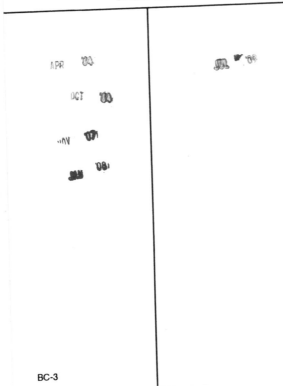

CANINE

ORTHOPEDICS

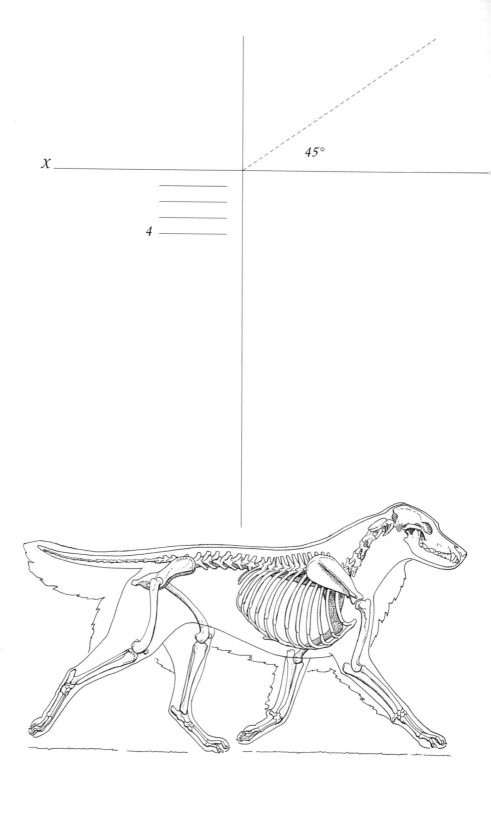

X

4

45°

CANINE
ORTHOPEDICS

ROBERT ROOKS, DVM, M.S.
DIPLOMATE AMERICAN BOARD OF VETERINARY PRACTITIONERS
DIPLOMATE AMERICAN COLLEGE OF VETERINARY SURGEONS
AND
CONNIE JANKOWSKI

WITH SPECIAL CONTRIBUTIONS BY
SUZANNA LEE, DVM

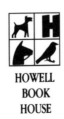

HOWELL
BOOK
HOUSE

Howell Book House
A Simon & Schuster Macmillan Company
1633 Broadway
New York, NY 10019

MACMILLAN is a registered trademark of Macmillan, Inc.

ISBN: 0-87605-720-2

Library of Congress Cataloging-in-Publication Data: CIP data available from Library of Congress upon request.

Manufactured in the United States of America

98 97 96   9 8 7 6 5 4 3 2 1

CONTENTS

ACKNOWLEDGMENTS

Dogs at work and dogs at play are works of art. The grace and agility demonstrated by a canine athlete rivals the beauty of a dancer practicing his or her art. A dog running full-out mimics the dancer executing a *grande jete;* each with legs extended to 180 degree angles—front legs forward, rear legs back. The arch of the neck and the straightness of the back reflect the intensity of the moment and produce the attitude that distinguishes the great ones.

We believe that a dog is a complete package and that all aspects of the dog's physical and mental health are interrelated. Often when we encounter behavior problems in dogs, we discover physical ailments. A painful dog cannot comfortably socialize, and the degree of pain suffered may relate to the degree of errant behavior. A dog in obvious pain is likely to bite anyone who comes near it. A dog in significant pain may become aggressive when handled. A dog with minor pain may be somewhat irritable. However, the correlation between pain and attitude cannot be denied—in pets or in people.

Some orthopedic problems are crippling. Some are mildly irritating, increasing in severity with the passage of time. Unfortunately, structural deformities occur quite frequently in dogs; however, most deformities are medically or surgically correctable. Not all dogs are Barishnicovs. Injuries and physical limitations prohibit many from dancing in the wind, but owner awareness can enable dogs to benefit from preventive and therapeutic treatments. Hopefully, this book will help to serve that goal.

I would like to thank the breeders and owners who have entrusted the care of their pets to me. For eighteen years of veterinary practice, I have been providing medical services to their special "kids." Their appreciation has been expressed in cards, letters, and photographs of the animals they love. I also thank my staff members for their contribution to the successful treatment and loving care they extend to our patients and their owners.

Calling attention to the importance of orthopedic soundness in dogs has long been the goal of the Orthopedic Foundation for Animals. The American Veterinary Medical Association, the American College of Veterinary Surgeons, the American Kennel Club, the Morris Animal

Foundation, and the veterinary teaching schools across the United States have been proactive in advancing the study of orthopedic disease in animals. Those associated with these groups can take great pride in their accomplishments as they charge forward to break new scientific grounds.

This book could not have been completed without the support of Suzanna Lee, DVM, and Linda Khachatoorian, RVT, who researched many of the chapters and whose involvement was essential to the completion of this project. We would also like to thank Vince Obsitnik, DVM, (spouse of Dr. Lee) of the Animal Medical Clinic in Peachtree City, Georgia, whose practice skills are among the best of veterinarians we have met.

Marcy Zingler, editor and accomplished canine authority, deserves heartfelt appreciation for her vision, her support of this project, and her patience in seeing it through. Monique Raymond, Stone Perales, and Chris Hoy lent their artistic flair with illustrations, and Kent Dannen's photos tell a story on their own.

Dog people, breeders, and other enthusiasts appreciate the beauty of a fine-moving dog and hold the key to improving pedigrees. We would like to thank breeders, judges, and the dog-mushing community, especially Susan Butcher, for sharing insights into the inner workings of the canine athlete, the character, the looseness.

Cecil Rooks (Bob's father) inspired this book in many ways. As a horse judge he was the best, and he taught others to find even the most subtle lamenesses. Watching an animal in motion, observing form during function, is the most important tool in analyzing structure and movement, even more diagnostic than palpation.

As with many published works about dogs, the spirits of beloved dogs inspired the meanings and the messages. Gone but not forgotten, their spirits live on. . .

INTRODUCTION

The body is a machine. In order for the machine to function efficiently, the parts must conform to the intended design of the entire unit.

Every dog's body has a specific design, and for a dog to perform the tasks intended, the body must operate efficiently. What is right for one dog may not be for another, but certain "manufacturing guidelines" apply to all dogs. A sports car may differ from a pickup truck, but all vehicles have axles and frames (chassis) that point all the wheels in the right direction. When a vehicle goes out of alignment, it fails to run smoothly, it burns more fuel, and it wears the tires quickly and unevenly. Dogs with misaligned bones move with an unsteady gait, expend needless energy, and wear down bone and soft tissue prematurely. As with any vehicle, problems associated with a dog's structure can be prevented, averted, or fixed before damage occurs.

The canine musculoskeletal system is the framework that supports the dog's other systems and enables the dog to move. Dogs cannot accompany us in the field or be desirable companions when they suffer chronic pain. How can we help our canine companions maximize their usefulness and enjoy their time with us? We must provide the essentials, including sound medical care.

A dog's inability to stand, walk, or run is shocking to observe. Certainly, these dogs experience great pain and reduced quality of life, and owners can recognize the need to seek veterinary care for their dogs. However, less severe lameness often goes undetected or is ignored. Owners then miss opportunities to secure medical intervention to correct problems before the condition worsens or causes irreversible damage.

As with all illnesses, early intervention in orthopedic disease produces the best chance for successful correction with the least amount of distress for the dog. Too often owners ignore lameness, "waiting for it to heal on its own." They deny the symptoms that plague dogs with degenerative processes, and they refuse surgical correction of "mildly dysplastic" dogs, not realizing that the longer the condition goes untreated, the worse the disease will progress.

A dog will compensate for a painful joint by distributing weight to other joints. Eventually the stress created by the extra weight bearing damages the once-healthy joints. Then the dog suffers from multiple orthopedic problems, and many require a series of surgeries to overcome the conditions.

Lameness can be attributed to three broad categories of causes: pain, mechanical restriction, and neurologic deficit. These categories can be further divided into common specific causes: congenital or acquired anomalies, trauma, hereditary or developmental conditions, metabolic disturbances, neoplasia, infection, and neurologic problems.

Damage to one part of this structure strains other parts, often producing severe damage to multiple sites. For example, a dog with hip dysplasia may alter its gait to relieve pain. The unnatural resultant gait shifts weight from one site to another. This shift can cause tearing of the anterior cruciate ligament (which runs through the rear knees), which in turn would require surgical repair.

Therefore, early detection and treatment of orthopedic abnormalities can alleviate pain in the affected joint and can prevent associated injuries as well. *Acute observation on the owner's part is crucial and can play a large role in successfully diagnosing problems.* The first sign of orthopedic abnormalities that dog owners may notice is an altered gait. A dog that limps, favors a leg, or hesitates to participate in activities calls attention to a problem. Owners should question odd behavior or changes in what is normal behavior for their dogs. Sometimes mild lameness goes undetected or is ignored, preventing early intervention and causing further degeneration.

Every dog should have an orthopedic evaluation during a regular veterinary examination. Consideration should be made to the conditions appropriate to the size and breed of dog, and owners should observe their dogs at home, noting unusual tendencies. The goal is to eliminate unsound dogs from breeding programs, to identify affected dogs early, and to obtain medical attention for those animals in need. Thereby, we eliminate pain and suffering and provide chances for full, enriched lifestyles.

Quality of life increases as pain decreases. The goals of general practitioners are to prevent pain and suffering and to relieve existing pain caused by disease or injury. Dog owners should seek preventive and (when appropriate) corrective measures to alleviate orthopedic abnormalities in their companion animals. When this occurs, dogs can reach their potentials as pets, companions, athletes, and workers.

GENERAL

CHAPTER 1

CONFORMATION AND BREEDING

"THE FIRST FRIEND"

by Rudyard Kipling

"When the Man waked up he said,
'What is Wild Dog doing here?'
And the Woman said,
'His name is not Wild Dog any more,
but the First Friend,
because he will be our friend
for always and always and always.'"

Nowhere is the human/animal bond stronger than between humans and dogs. The relationship that evolved through centuries of codependency has withstood the test of time. People and dogs have worked together and played together, developing the trust and love that family members share. However, our fascination with dogs has not been an entirely beneficial experience for the dog. To see the effects of selective breeding, we must study what occurs in nature.

Throughout the world, people have observed packs of free-roaming dogs, both urban and rural, that consist of cast-off pets and feral-born strays. The dogs have been allowed to interbreed and reproduce indiscriminately. Consistent from location to location is the emergence of a recognizable "type" of pack dog.

Medium-sized, shorthaired, medium-boned, brown dogs have been observed in every setting. The dogs, who were created without human interference, exhibit the same characteristics of the dogs thought to have been man's first companions. The dogs seem to be remarkably healthy, supposedly owing to the survival of the fittest theories, and also appear to be consistently free of orthopedic disease. However, since these animals are rarely tested, we do not know for sure to what extent this may be true.

However, because people have varying tastes and seek different qualities in companion animals, we have created a diversity of styles to

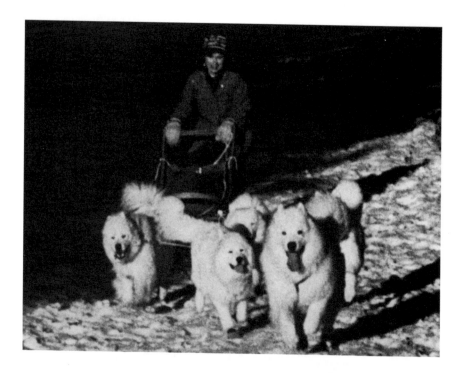

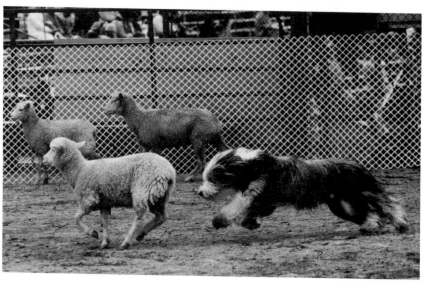

Because purebred dogs have been selectively bred for various characteristics, breeders must take caution to produce sound animals to preserve their given breed. The Samoyed dog team can pull a sled, and this Bearded Collie covers ground to do her job, herding sheep, as intended.   *Photos by Kent and Donna Dannen*

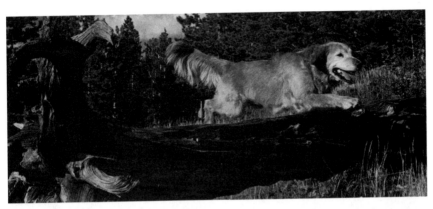

The Golden Retriever can work in the field. *Photo by Kent and Donna Dannen*

meet various needs and preferences in dogs through centuries of selective breeding. From the tiny Chihuahua to the regal Irish Wolfhound, all dogs relate back to that ancestral, feral dog. Dogs most removed from the ancestral dog have experienced the greatest degree of deviation from the norm, sometimes to the dogs' regret.

The laws of genetics dictate that focusing on one direction of body form creates a decline in supporting structure in another area. Modifications in body type have enabled the canine species to perform specific functions. A skeletal analysis and study of the musculoskeletal framework demonstrate the multitude of tasks that have evolved for canine companions. However, disregard for structural balance has led to an increase in orthopedic disease.

EVALUATING CANINE CONFORMATION

Before buying a dog or choosing breeding stock, pay careful attention to the dogs' structure and movement. Learn to assess a dog's balance. The canine body should be viewed for symmetry, size, and shape. Both the relation of each portion to the others and the overall appearance should be pleasing to the eye of the beholder. The ambiguity of this statement is necessary due to the various traits desired. What is acceptable in one breed may be obviously unacceptable in another. Even within breeds, conformation differences occur based on the strength of various bloodlines. Individual conformation is an inherited trait that cannot be altered.

Conformation balance is often a common denominator among various breed Standards. Drawing a line from the point of the elbow to the top of the shoulder and another from the cranial aspect of the stifle to the cranial aspect of the hip, the body can be divided into three

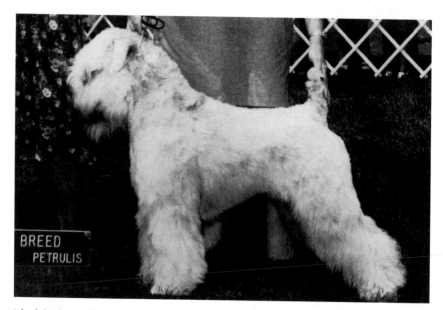

BREED
PETRULIS

Ideal limb conformation includes proper length of the bones as well as proper angulation. Dog show judges closely evaluate the "balance" demonstrated in each entry, as dictated by the appropriate breed Standard. This Soft Coated Wheaten Terrier shows proper type and balance.   *Photo courtesy of Carla Cohen*

equal parts. A horizontal line drawn between the heads of the femur and humerus roughly divides the body into halves. Axial alignment is evaluated by drawing a visual line from the center of the shoulder down the center of the back to the base of the tail. Marked differences in bone length can cause unequal stress on joints and potential orthopedic problems.

Another contributor to stress of the musculoskeletal system is abnormal limb angulation. Just as alignment is important to the efficient operation of a vehicle, proper bone alignment allows a body to move efficiently, without wearing down the joint structures.

How does alignment affect movement? For example, a straight shoulder leads to decreased angulation and shorter stride with more steps needed to cover given distances. Slightened angles of the stifle and hock also reduce range of motion and the ability to cover ground with each stride. Reduced or excessive angulation also creates stress on the joint surfaces, causing abnormalities, ligament degeneration, or secondary degenerative joint disease.

An area for potential imbalance deals with weight distribution. The normal standing weight distribution in the dog is for 60% of the body weight to be supported by both front limbs and 40% supported by the

Good front assembly.

Front is east/west.
Toes point out to the side.

Toes point inward.

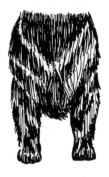
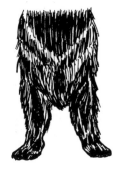
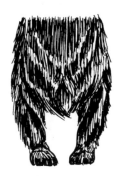

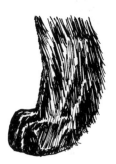
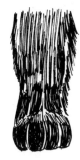

Good, tight, "cat" foot.
(Side and Front view)

Weak, "hare" feet, with
splayed toes.

Broken down foot with
weak pasterns.

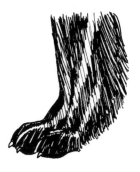
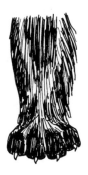
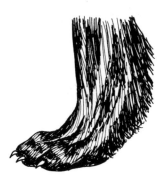

A strong front indicates proper function in the shoulders, wrists, and elbows. Alignment can be evaluated with the dog moving or standing.

Illustrations by Monique Raymond

Good rear, hocks are
parallel to each other.

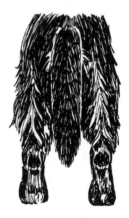

Hocks point inward, known
as cow hocks.

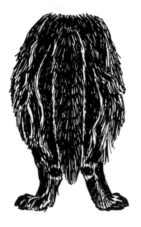

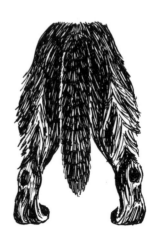

Hocks point outward, or
bowlegged.

The hips, knees, and hocks should be symmetrical; observe the dog standing and moving.

rear limbs. The center of gravity is balanced in the standing animal between the two front limbs and one hind limb. Movement of one of the front limbs causes a necessary shift of the center of gravity toward the hind limbs.

Biomechanical forces change weight support when there is an increase in speed. The physiological force that occurs when the foot makes contact with the ground is influenced by weight bearing, muscle contraction, and body acceleration. With acceleration, the ground force may increase to more than five times the normal body weight. Large weight bearing loads are transmitted to the bones through the joints. The main function of the pasterns (carpal joints) is to diffuse this force through the front limbs. Proper conformation supports the use of the forelimbs. The hind limbs function as a driving train, affecting the fore-limbs as well as propelling the body forward.

CONFORMATIONAL ABNORMALITIES

Conformation abnormalities, such as when the angulation of the limbs or postural stance is asymmetrical, can be congenital or acquired. Congenital deformities associated with hip dysplasia include subluxa-tion, which is seen with an increase or decrease of angulation of the femoral neck and shaft. Acquired abnormalities may include nutrition-al bone disease or fractures that have healed as a malunion (incorrect alignment of fracture fragments).

Dwarfism in dogs can be a desired or undesired inherited trait. Many breeds have been created by breeding individuals displaying dwarfism, an abnormal growth of cartilage (chondrodysplasia). The Bulldog, Pekingese, Basset Hound, and Dachshund are examples of breeds that have been selected for the stunting or bowing of limbs, deviation of feet, and changes in joint surfaces. This stunting was a con-scious selection of an otherwise abnormal form to serve a functional purpose. However, dwarfism occurs in some breeds as an *undesirable* inherited trait.

Different aspects of dwarfism can be demonstrated in various forms. Achondroplasia is a cartilage growth failure in young dogs. Faulty growth plate formation (enchondrodystrophy) may be consid-ered a form of chondrodysplasia. Abnormal skeletal bone formation with increased areas of bone density is another type of chondrodys-plastic dwarfism known as epiphyseal dysplasia. It may involve the entire skeleton or only a portion. Insufficient amounts of growth hor-mone can cause pituitary dwarfism. This disease delays the closure of the normal growth plates while maintaining the soft puppy hair coat.

FORM AND FUNCTION

For each function that canine companions have been called upon to perform, there are specific body types best suited to those tasks.

The limbs should be well suited to the breed type, as well as body height, depth, and length. The limbs act as vertical struts, similar to the supporting structures of a bridge. The head and tail serve as the bal-

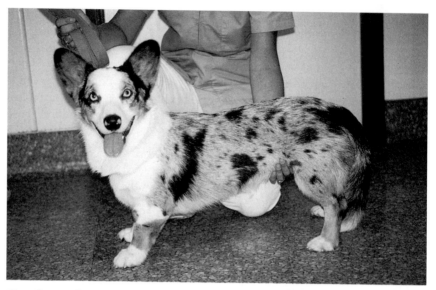

Dwarfism in dogs can be a desired (as illustrated by this Cardigan Welsh Corgi) or undesired inherited trait. Many breeds have been created by breeding individuals displaying dwarfism, an abnormal growth of cartilage (chondrodysplasia).

ancing arms for the ends of the bridge. Ideal limb conformation includes proper length of bones as well as proper angulation.

Bone length varies with breed type. For example, the racing sled dog, a highly specialized canine athlete, is considered ideal when the four major bones (scapula, humerus, pelvis, and femur) are close to equal in length. To evaluate a dog, measure the bones and compare. Differences in bone length can cause unequal biomechanical stress on the joints and potential orthopedic problems. Although your dog may not be a sled dog, it is important that the bones are symmetrical (the right and left sides equal) but not necessarily all equal in length (the scapula and pelvis tend to be shorter than the femur and humerus). A lack of symmetry from side to side can also cause unequal stress and problems.

Skeletal muscles make up almost half of the adult dog's body weight. Skeletal muscles allow for voluntary body movement while adapting and responding to work and exercise. Muscles can be classi-fied as aerobic or anaerobic and will develop according to function. For example, if a muscle must bear a large load, it will respond by grow-ing larger and stronger. In response to lighter, more repetitive work or exercise, the muscles adapt by increasing their ability to produce the energy needed for the sustained activity. Heavier muscles contract more slowly (muscle-bound) than light muscles. There is a fine dis-tinction between over- and under-muscled dogs.

The angle of the pelvis partially determines the ability of the hind limbs to extend backward. Quick turning, heavy pulling, or running uphill are all benefited by steep angulation of the pelvis (45 degrees off horizontal). Stifle angulation determines how easily dogs can pull (harness dogs). Straighter stifles hinder jumping, whereas a stifle with a greater bend creates longer rear reach and greater flexibility. Well-bent stifles enhance speed, jumping, and go-to-ground capabilities in dogs. The length of the hocks has an effect on function, since long hocks are beneficial for initial speed and shorter hocks provide endurance and power.

Foot conformation is directly related to function as well. Round, compact feet (cat feet) are best suited for endurance. Oval shaped feet

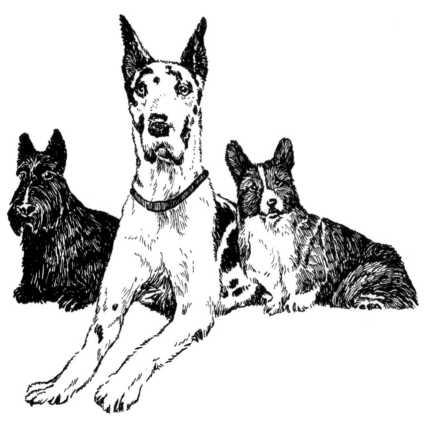

Every breed is governed by a Standard, which details the physical and temperament details of the ideal representative of that breed. Otherwise, a German Shepherd Dog would soon look and act like a Belgian Malinois. A Tibetan Terrier and a Lhasa Apso would be alike. Not only would appearance be diluted and compromised, so would function and ability to perform the appropriate tasks of the breed.   *Illustration by Chris Hoy*

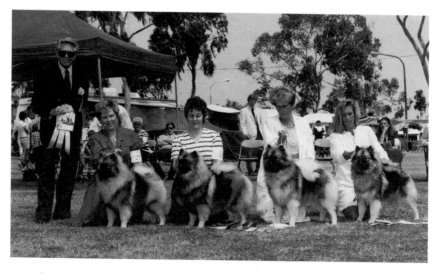

Complying with the Standard and breeding to avoid conformational abnormalities are the goals of responsible breeders and help increase the odds of producing sound puppies. This six to nine month puppy bitch class at a Southern California dog show allows breeders to measure the quality of their puppies against others.

Photo by Missy Yuhl

have slightly elongated third digits, representing a compromise between endurance and a high initial speed or jumping ability. Hare shaped feet are represented by dog breeds that were developed for high initial speed and jumping. Webbed feet increase surface space while providing better movement through water, mud, or snow. Foot shape can be affected by heredity, lack of exercise during development, improper nutrition, and improper ground surface during growth.

PUREBRED DOGS

Because purebred dogs have been selectively bred for various characteristics, breeders must take caution to produce sound animals. Each breed is governed by a Standard, which details the physical and temperamental details of the ideal representative of that breed, and breeders strive to produce puppies that conform to that Standard. Less than perfect conformation is a factor in the development of orthopedic diseases.

To know what is abnormal, you have to know what is normal. The physical description of breeds varies greatly. Each breed Standard should specify the ideal height, length of the back, carriage of tail, and angulation of the limbs. Furthermore, the Standard will identify the appropriate gait for a breed and the placement of feet when moving and standing still. What is correct gait? It varies from breed to breed. Most sighthounds single track, but herding dogs do not. The rolling gait of an Old English Sheepdog is desirable for that breed, but unacceptable for most others. Complying with the Standard by breeding to avoid

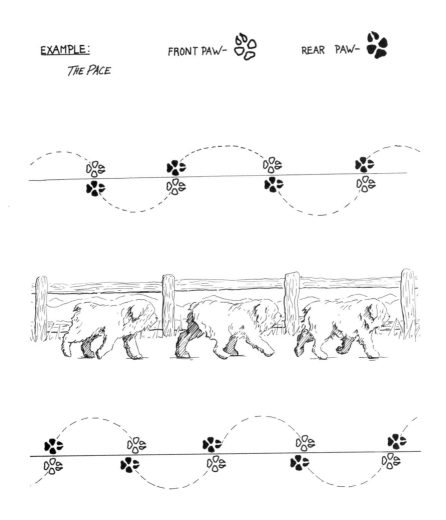

The Old English Sheepdog is, according to the Standard, "A strong, compact, square, balanced dog . . . . He is thickset, muscular, and able-bodied . . . fit for the demanding tasks required of a shepherd's or drover's dog. Therefore soundness is of the greatest importance. When trotting, movement is free and powerful, seemingly effortless with good reach and drive, and covering maximum ground with minimum steps. [The dogs are] very elastic at a gallop, [and they] may amble or pace at slower speeds."   *Illustration by Monique Raymond*

conformational abnormalities is the goal of responsible breeders and helps increase the odds for producing sound puppies.

Dog shows are held to evaluate dogs' closeness to the Standard. While grooming, handling skills, and presentation may influence a dog's chances at winning, structure and movement play a great role in success or failure. Dog show judges perform physical assessments of the dogs in the ring. They observe the dogs for overall symmetry, they feel the dogs, and they evaluate angulation, shoulder layback, and length of neck. They observe the dog moving away (view of the rear), moving laterally from the side (for view of reach and drive, the topline [back], and neck carriage), and moving toward the judge (view of the front assembly). The judge can assess fluidity of movement (as appropriate to the breed), reach and drive, placement of feet, and ease of movement.

The evaluation performed at a dog show is much like that performed during an orthopedic examination, and dog show judges, breeders, and

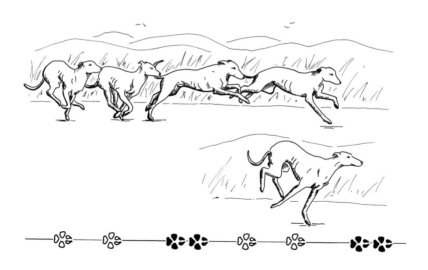

According to the American Kennel Club Standard for the Whippet, "Gait [should be] low, free moving, and smooth, with reach in the forequarters and strong drive in the hindquarters. The dog has great freedom of action when viewed from the side; the forelegs move forward close to the ground to give a long low reach; the hind legs have strong propelling power. When moving and viewed from the front or rear, legs should turn neither in nor out, nor should feet cross or interfere with each other. Lack of front reach or rear drive, or a short, hackney gait with high wrist action, should be strictly penalized. Crossing in front or moving too closely should be strictly penalized." *Illustration by Monique Raymond*

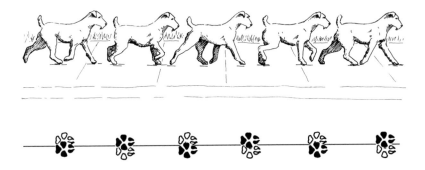

The AKC Standard for the Wire Fox Terrier describes gait in great detail: "The movement or action is the crucial test of conformation. The terrier's legs should be carried straight forward while traveling, the forelegs hanging perpendicular and swinging parallel to the sides, like the pendulum of a clock. The principal propulsive power is furnished by the hind legs, perfection of action being found in the terrier possessing long thighs and muscular second thighs well bent at the stifles, which admit of a strong forward thrust or 'snatch' of the hocks. When approaching, the forelegs should form a continuation of the straight of the front, the feet being the same distance apart as the elbows. When stationary it is often difficult to determine whether a dog is slightly out at shoulder, but directly when he moves, the defect— if it exists—becomes more apparent, the forefeet having a tendency to cross, 'weave,' or 'dish.' When on the contrary, the dog is tied at the shoulder, the tendency of the feet is to move wider apart with a sort of paddling action. When the hocks are turned in—cow-hocks—the stifles and feet are turned outwards, resulting in a serious loss of propulsive power. When the hocks are turned outwards the tendency of the hind feet is to cross, resulting in an ungainly waddle."

Illustration by Monique Raymond

handlers are often quite adept at identifying orthopedic abnormalities. In fact, dog show fanciers may be more skilled than some medical personnel in observing dogs and detecting lameness.

Professionals interested in the performance aspects of dogs are also astutely aware of orthopedic defects. A dog cannot work the field, herd sheep, or protect and serve in a law enforcement capacity if it is lame and in pain. Dogs that compete in Obedience Trials, Frisbee competitions, Field Trials, or Agility competitions cannot respond with the energy needed if they are not physically fit. Heightened awareness of lameness comes from observation, comparison, and consideration of functional needs.

BREEDING

The goal in breeding a litter of puppies should be threefold. Breeders should strive to:

1. Produce dogs that are physically equipped to perform the function intended.
2. Produce dogs that are mentally sound.
3. Ensure that these dogs go to homes fit to house them.

Often, people rely on "papers" to ensure quality in the puppies they buy. However, *registration papers in no way guarantee the quality of a dog,* but rather, registration papers merely acknowledge that the litter of puppies is out of registered parents, recorded by an organization such as the American Kennel Club. The quality of dogs varies from breeder to breeder, and attention to orthopedic soundness is essential to a reputable breeder.

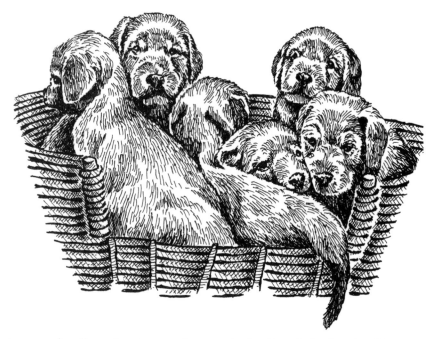

Anyone who allows dogs to reproduce can be legally called a breeder. However, the term carries many levels open to interpretation. Golden Retrievers are very popular, therefore the demand for puppies has encouraged many novices to breed their dogs. However, quality (in physical appearance and underlying structure) varies greatly among Goldens you see on the street.   *Illustration by Chris Hoy*

WHAT IS A DOG BREEDER?

Technically, anyone owning a female who reproduces is called a breeder. However, the term carries many levels of interpretation. For practical considerations, we generally categorize breeders in four categories:

1. *The Accidental Breeder.* Through neglect (a subtle form of abuse), accidental breeders allow their dogs to randomly mate and reproduce. Many of these dogs are mixed breeds, and "breeders" often experience great difficulty finding homes for these dogs.
2. *The Commercial Breeder.* People who supply puppies for retail sales often seek quantity over quality. They support themselves with mass sales of various dogs to distributors who resell them to commercial dog-selling establishments (often to pet stores). The dog buyer (or consumer) is so far removed from the "breeder" of the dog that important questions about the dog's genetic makeup and early socialization cannot be asked. The mass-producing "breeder" rarely performs screening (such as x-raying for hip dysplasia), rarely knows the ancestors of the dogs (let alone the medical histories), and rarely (if ever) follows up to track the development of the puppies.
3. *The Backyard Breeder.* Owners of "nice pets" often receive favorable comments from friends about their beautiful dogs. Owners of purebred pets hear about the opportunity to earn extra money selling puppies. This encourages genuinely nice people to dabble in the business of breeding dogs.

    These pet owners often start with dogs acquired from people who have no experience in breeding dogs, or else they would have been advised about the complications associated with dog breeding. So the breeding stock they start with may be inferior.

    Rarely do backyard breeders perform genetic screening, nor do they have information about the genetic background of the dogs they breed. Furthermore, the selection of a stud dog is left to chance. The dog that lives down the street, is owned by a relative, or is advertised in the local newspaper is usually the stud chosen— without regard to quality.
4. *The Responsible Breeder.* These people breed dogs for a purpose. Responsible breeders study the breed of choice by attending dog events, such as dog shows or field trials; and they compare notes with other breeders to obtain the necessary information for making good choices in selecting breeding stock.

    Responsible breeders may raise dogs for a functional need, such as herding dogs, sporting dogs, or sled dogs; or their main goal in breeding may be to produce companion animals. However, all responsible breeders strive to eliminate structural weaknesses from their breeding programs. Responsible breeders screen their dogs for congenital defects before they are bred.

In respect to orthopedic soundness, responsible breeders routinely test their breeding stock using Orthopedic Foundation for Animals (OFA) and PennHIP® procedures. Furthermore, dogs may be tested for von Willebrand's disease and hypothyroidism, which can influence soundness. Breeds predisposed to other diseases should be screened for the conditions that affect the breed. Veterinarians can assess and certify dogs found clear of such conditions as slipping stifles, progressive retinal atrophy (PRA, a disease of the eye), and congenital heart defects.

GENETICS

Living beings are the product of their genetic makeup. Whether a breeder is conscious of the subtleties of genetic engineering, the puppies produced reflect a breeder's knowledge, effort, and ethics—or lack thereof.

Planning a litter requires breeders to consider principles of genetics. And although puppies *can* be born without the benefit of considering genetic value, puppies should *not* be conceived without this safeguard. Although problems can arise in the best-planned litters, the chances for producing unhealthy puppies are minimized when the breeder screens the breeding stock—and the generations of dogs that appear in the dogs' pedigrees—for genetic flaws.

At the moment of conception every dog acquires the features it will display and it will pass to future generations through its genes. Each puppy receives genes from its father and its mother, and the traits the puppy will display usually depend upon expression of dominant characteristics. How do you track the genes in a breeding line?

Some genetic qualities are easier to trace than others. For example, eye color can be documented and studied. Let us use eye color to describe the basic principles of dominant/recessive genetics. Brown eyes are a dominant feature and blue eyes are recessive. When a baby receives a blue-eye gene from one parent and a brown-eye gene from the other, the baby will have brown eyes, although he or she will carry one brown-eye gene and one blue-eye gene, and either can be passed to future generations.

Therefore, a brown-eyed animal could parent a blue-eyed child, if both parents carry at least one blue gene and the child inherits blue genes from each parent. A blue-eyed animal can parent a brown-eyed child if the other parent is brown eyed and passes on a brown gene.

In respect to orthopedics, an animal's predisposition to disease is hereditary, reflective of the animal's genetic makeup. Complex traits,

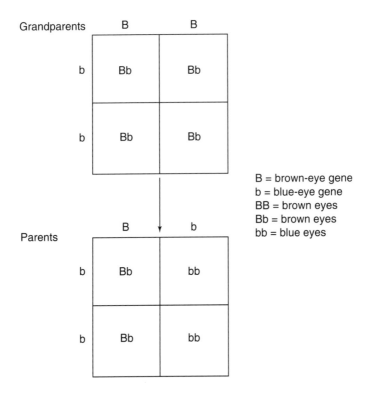

B = brown-eye gene
b = blue-eye gene
BB = brown eyes
Bb = brown eyes
bb = blue eyes

such as bone structure and temperament, are more complicated to monitor than eye color. These traits are controlled by multiple pairs of genes that together produce the traits expressed in the dog. The term additive genes is given to sets of genes that combine to establish a complex quality, such as hip structure.

Traits established by a single gene pair are easy to manipulate, and orchestrated changes can be witnessed in a single generation. Complex qualities involve many gene pairs and are therefore more difficult to effect. Planned changes to a complex quality in a line, such as the elimination of hip dysplasia, often take several generations to achieve.

Therefore, in the process of elimination, many puppies will demonstrate the undesirable trait, such as dysplasia, when known carriers of the disease are bred—even when long-term planning is to eliminate the disease. Ethical considerations dictate that many animals be eliminated from breeding programs, even though they may have numerous good qualities, in order to avoid producing animals with serious medical defects.

Puppy and adult dog buyers must seek to purchase from responsible breeders. Because dysplasia is the most troubling of orthopedic concerns, buyers are often cautioned to be sure the sire and dam of a

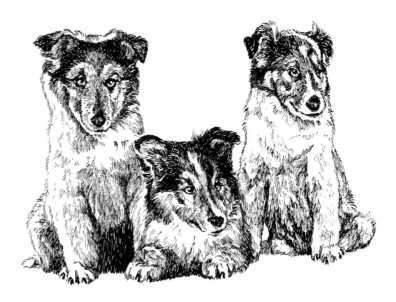

Living beings are the product of their genetic makeup. The genetic variances are obvious in puppies in some litters, others are very difficult to see—except by a trained eye. The Shelties are different in size, sex, and coloring.   *Illustration by Chris Hoy*

litter have been x-rayed and are clear of hip and elbow dysplasia, but few pet owners understand the significance of this recommendation.

Dysplasia is not the only concern for responsible dog breeders. Luxating patellas, spinal malformation, and other growth related diseases should also be addressed by the breeder and the prospective buyer to strengthen the total dog. Beware of the breeder that is reluctant to discuss diseases, or who claims to have perfect puppies. Honest willingness to discuss the health of a litter is a good sign in a breeder.

Breeding dogs should not be a passing fancy, but rather the product of years of studying a breed and knowledge about the dogs and bitches in your breeding program. In addition to a display case full of dog show ribbons and trophies, responsible breeders can display their knowledge of their dogs' genetic histories. Only then can the quality of dogs produced in each generation improve.

CHAPTER 2

BREED PREDISPOSITIONS

Are purebred dogs at greater risk of developing orthopedic problems than mixed-breed dogs? *Orthopedic problems can affect dogs of any breed or mix.*

The unintentional pairing of recessive genes can produce orthopedic abnormalities, and the chances increase as the gene pool gets smaller. All dogs should be carefully evaluated prior to selection for breeding. Orthopedic diseases and other genetic problems should be strongly considered when animals are to be bred, *including* problems with the dogs in their pedigrees and dogs produced by close relatives. If a breeder cannot tell you anything about a puppy's grandparents or half-siblings, you should question the breeder's depth of knowledge.

Purebred dogs have been studied a great deal; mixes generally have not. Patterns of disease transmission have been identified in some breeds and lines, but because of a lack of sufficient data, such patterns cannot be traced in mixes. For this reason, much of our discussion revolves around purebreds. Generally speaking, large and giant dogs experience a higher incidence of growth-related lameness as well as hip dysplasia. Heavy, large-boned dogs commonly stress the joints, traumatizing the joint structures. Rottweilers, Labrador Retrievers, and American Pit Bull Terriers are prime candidates for rupturing the cruciate ligaments in the knee. Small dogs are prone to problems in the knees. Medium-sized dogs have the fewest incidences of orthopedic disease, but any dog can be affected.

The list of orthopedic problems provided here includes most American Kennel Club breeds and is organized by Group to facilitate comparison of similar type dogs. Please note that the breeds are arranged by strict alphabetical order within the Group. Some breeds have been omitted because data has not been reported about those dogs. Statements made about a breed's predisposition to disease must be regarded as generalizations, *not* absolutes. Data collected about the various breeds reflects printed literature and personal observations. While we await scientifically controlled and documented studies on each breed, trends can be noted by breeders and veterinarians and can produce generalized statements about a various breed's likelihood to suffer a specific condition.

The information may be useful to breeders in selecting breeding pairs, to puppy buyers in selecting a pet or show prospect, and to pet owners in assuring that their dogs receive proper screening and subsequent treatment for affected dogs. Prevention is the best cure for disease, but early detection provides the greatest number of treatment options.

SPORTING DOGS

Brittanys   Patella luxation; Hip dysplasia

Chesapeake Bay Retrievers   Hip dysplasia; Elbow dysplasia

Clumber Spaniels   Hip dysplasia

Cocker Spaniels (American)   Hip dysplasia; IVD (intervertebral disk disease); Patella luxation, either medial or lateral; Elbow dysplasia; Thyroid disorders; Neoplasias; Anury (no tail, no caudal vertebrae); Brachury (short tail)

Curly-Coated Retrievers   Thyroid disorders; Calcium metabolic disorders; Juvenile osteoporosis

English Cocker Spaniels   Swimmers syndrome (i.e. the inability to stand at four to six weeks of age)

English Setters   Hip dysplasia; Neoplasias

English Springer Spaniels   Hip dysplasia; Myasthenia gravis

Field Spaniels   Thyroid disorders; Hip dysplasia

Flat-Coated Retrievers   Hip dysplasia; Patella luxation; Neoplasias

German Shorthaired Pointers   Pannus; Neoplasias

German Wirehaired Pointers   Hip dysplasia; Toe fractures

Golden Retrievers   Hip dysplasia (very high incidence); Elbow dysplasia; OCD (osteochondritis dissecans) of elbow; Muscular dystrophy; Thyroid disorders; Neoplasias

Gordon Setters   Hip dysplasia; Thyroid disorders

Irish Setters   Generalized myopathy (i.e. stiff gait and other difficulties); Carpal (pastern) luxation; OCD—especially in knees and shoulders; Metabolic bone disease; Neoplasias; Thyroid disorders; Hip dysplasia

Irish Water Spaniels   Hip dysplasia

Labrador Retrievers   Carpal (pastern) luxation associated with Hemophilia A; Dwarfism associated with retinal dysplasia; Muscle mass deficiency; Deficiency of type II muscle fibers; Hip dysplasia; Elbow dysplasia; Muscular dystrophy; Thyroid disorders

Pointers   Neurotropic osteopathy; Low sensitivity in distal limbs; Demyelination in spinal cord; self-mutilation; Toe gnawing; Neuromuscular atrophy; Hip dysplasia; Dwarfism

Sussex Spaniels   IVD (intervertebral disk disease)

Vizslas   Hip dysplasia

Weimaraners   Spinal dysraphism (crouching stance, abduction of one leg, and hopping gait); Hip dysplasia; Myasthenia gravis; Neoplasias; Elbow dysplasia; Dwarfism

Welsh Springer Spaniels   Hip dysplasia; Thyroid disorders

Wirehaired Pointing Griffons   Hip dysplasia

HOUNDS

Afghan Hounds   Elbow dysplasia; Malformation of articular surfaces of proximal radius and ulna; Thyroid disorders

American Foxhounds   Spinal osteochondrosis (affects the ability to run)

Basenjis   Hip dysplasia

Bassset Hounds   Vertebral deformity with pressure necrosis results from anomaly of third cervical vertebra; Achondroplasia (foreleg lameness caused by anatomical irregularity; cartilage of growth plate grows in irregular directions and is scant); OCD (shoulder); Osteodystrophy; Radial carpal joint irregularity; Patella luxation, medial or lateral that produces lameness at four to six months of age; IVD (intervertebral disk disease); Panosteitis

Beagles   Hip dysplasia; Epiphyseal dysplasia; IVD

Black and Tan Coonhounds   Hip dysplasia (high incidence); Polyradiculoneuritis; Coondog paralysis

Bloodhounds   Hip dysplasia; Elbow dysplasia

Borzois   Thyroid disorders

Dachshunds   IVD; Osteoporosis clinically similar to swimmers, with radiographs showing dense bones and abnormal bone resorption; UAP (ununited anconeal process); Patella luxation; Achondroplasia; Thyroid disorders

English Foxhounds   Osteochondrosis of the spine; Intervertebral disk disease

Greyhounds   Short spine

Harriers   Hip dysplasia

Irish Wolfhounds   Elbow hygroma; Hip dysplasia; Elbow dysplasia; Metabolic bone disease; UAP; Neoplasias

Otterhounds   Hip dysplasia (high incidence); Elbow dysplasia

Petit Basset Griffon Vendeens   Hip dysplasia

Pharaoh Hounds   Medial patella luxation

Rhodesian Ridgebacks   Cervical vertebral deformity; Hip dysplasia; Lumbosacral transitional vertebrae

Salukis   Hip dysplasia

Scottish Deerhounds   OCD

Whippets   Toe injuries

WORKING DOGS

Akitas   Juvenile polyarthritis causing incapacitating pain and fever; Hip dysplasia; Elbow dysplasia; Thyroid disorders

Alaskan Malamutes   Hip dysplasia; Chondrodysplasia, a dwarfism associated with anemia that produces stunted growth in the forelegs, lateral deviation of the foot, carpal enlargement, bowing of forelegs, and a sloping topline; Polyneuropathy, an hereditary progressive muscle weakness

Bernese Mountain Dogs   Hip dysplasia (very high incidence); Elbow dysplasia; Neoplasias

Boxers   Neoplasias; Intervertebral disk degeneration; Cardiomyopathy

Bullmastiffs   Hip dysplasia; Elbow dysplasia; Cervical vertebral malformation; UAP

Doberman Pinschers   Wobblers syndrome; Polyostotic fibrous dysplasia (osteophytes and cysts form in distal metaphyses of ulna and radius); Neoplasias; Elbow dysplasia

Giant Schnauzers   Hip dysplasia (high incidence); OCD; Thyroid disorders

Great Danes   Wobblers syndrome; Stockard's paralysis (Preganglionic sympathetic degeneration onset at about three months of age); Cervical calcinosis circumscripta; OCD; Metabolic bone disease; Neoplasias; Elbow dysplasia; UAP

Great Pyrenees   Hip dysplasia; Patella luxation; Swimmers syndrome (the inability to stand at four to six weeks of age); Brittle bone syndrome; UAP

Greater Swiss Mountain Dogs   Hip dysplasia; OCD

Komondorok   Hip dysplasia

Kuvaszok   Hip dysplasia

Mastiffs   Hip dysplasia; Elbow dysplasia

Newfoundlands   Hip dysplasia (high incidence); Elbow dysplasia; UAP

Portuguese Water Dogs   Hip dysplasia

Rottweilers   Hip dysplasia (high incidence); Elbow dysplasia; OCD; Muscular dystrophy

St. Bernards   Stockard's paralysis; Neoplasias; Hip dysplasia (high incidence); Metabolic bone disease; Elbow dysplasia; OCD; Wobblers syndrome

Samoyeds   Hip dysplasia; Dwarfism; Muscular dystrophy

Siberian Huskies   Hip dysplasia

Standard Schnauzers   Hip dysplasia; Thyroid disorders

TERRIERS

Airedale Terriers   Hip dysplasia; Trembling hindquarters seen after six months of age; Thyroid disorders

American Staffordshire Terriers   Ruptured cruciate ligament (very common)

Australian Terriers   Legg-Calves Perthes disease; Patella luxation

Border Terriers   Patella luxation; Hip dysplasia

Bull Terriers   None recorded in veterinary literature

Cairn Terriers   Patella luxation; Legg-Calves Perthes disease

Dandie Dinmont Terriers   IVD; Achondroplasia; Patella luxation, either medial or lateral; Hip dysplasia; Shoulder luxation; Elbow dysplasia; Neoplasias

Fox Terriers (Smooth and Wire)   Shoulder dislocation; Legg-Calves Perthes disease; Myasthenia gravis

Irish Terriers   Muscular dystrophy

Kerry Blue Terriers   UAP

Lakeland Terriers   UAP; Legg-Calves Perthes disease.

Manchester Terriers (Standard and Toy)   Legg-Calves Perthes disease

Miniature Schnauzers   Legg-Calves Perthes disease; Muscular dystrophy

Scottish Terriers   Dwarfism; Scottie cramp, characterized by rigidity of limbs with dog recovering in 30 seconds; Thyroid disorders; Elbow dysplasia; IVD

Sealyham Terriers   IVD

Skye Terriers   Thyroid disorders

Soft Coated Wheaten Terriers   Hip dysplasia

Staffordshire Bull Terriers   None recorded in veterinary literature

Welsh Terriers   Medial patella luxation

West Highland White Terriers   Legg-Calves Perthes disease; Patella luxation; Hip dysplasia

TOY DOGS

Affenpinschers   Patella luxation, either medial or lateral; Legg-Calves Perthes disease

Brussels Griffons   Shoulder dislocation

Cavalier King Charles Spaniels   Patella luxation; Episodic weakness and collapse, a rare, inherited disorder

Chihuahuas (Long and Smooth coats)   Shoulder dislocation; Patella luxation, medial or lateral; Hypoplasia of dens, which produces atlantoaxial subluxation, causing neck pain and quadriplegia

Chinese Cresteds   Medial patella luxation; Legg-Calves Perthes disease

English Toy Spaniels (Blenheim/Prince Charles and King Charles/Ruby)   Patella luxation, medial or lateral can occur with medial the most common; Congenital Femoral Shift

Italian Greyhounds   Predisposed to forelimb fractures

Japanese Chin   Dwarfism

Maltese   Patella luxation

Miniature Pinschers   Shoulder dislocation; Legg-Calves Perthes disease; Epiphyseal dysplasia; Decreased long-bone growth; Osteopenia

Papillons   Patella luxation

Pekingese   Hypoplasia of dens (Odontoid Process, an atlantoaxial subluxation, causes neck pain and quadriplegia); IVD; Swimmers syndrome; Atypical pannus; Legg-Calves Perthes disease

Pomeranians   Patella luxation, either medial or lateral; Dwarfism; Hypoplasia of dens, atlantoaxial subluxation

Poodles (Toy)   Dwarfism; Atypical pannus; Patella luxation; IVD; Legg-Calves Perthes disease; Thyroid disorders; Neoplasias

Pugs   Atypical pannus; Legg-Calves Perthes disease; Patella luxation, medial

Shih Tzus   Dwarfism; Patella luxation

Silky Terriers   Patella luxation; Legg-Calves Perthes disease

Yorkshire Terriers   Patella luxation, medial or lateral; Hypoplasia of dens, which produces atlantoaxial subluxation, neck pain, and quadriplegia; Legg-Calves Perthes disease

NON-SPORTING DOGS

American Eskimo Dogs   Hip dysplasia

Bichons Frises   Patella luxation

Boston Terriers   Neoplasias; Patella luxation, either medial or lateral; Swimmers syndrome, the inability to stand at four to six weeks; Vertebral abnormalities

Bulldogs   Spina bifida, caused by ununited neural arches; Neoplasias; Swimmers syndrome, the inability to stand at four to six weeks; Hip dysplasia; Elbow dysplasia; Flaccid shoulder joints; Thyroid disorders; Vertebral abnormalities

Chinese Shar-Peis   Patella luxation; Hip dysplasia; Elbow dysplasia; Swollen hock syndrome

Chow Chows   Hip dysplasia; Elbow dysplasia

Dalmatians   Muscular dystrophy

Finnish Spitz   Patella luxation

French Bulldogs   Hemivertebrae, which is the asymmetric abnormal development of vertebrae, resulting in scoliosis and crowding of one half of the body, producing a wedge-shape. It often results in neonatal death or spinal cord compression in older puppies

Keeshonds   Thyroid and other endocrine disorders, primary hyperparathyroidism in older dogs; Patella luxation; Hip dysplasia; Neoplasias

Lhasa Apsos   Patella luxation, either medial or lateral; Hip dysplasia

Poodles (Miniature)   Dwarfism; Hypoplasia of dens; Atypical pannus; Patella luxation; Shoulder luxation; IVD; Legg-Calves Perthes disease; Thyroid disorders; Neoplasias; Epiphyseal dysplasia.

Poodles (Standard)   Osteogenesis imperfecta, shown in deficient bone growth resulting in frequent fractures; Atypical pannus; Neoplasias; Hip dysplasia; Thyroid disorders

Schipperkes   Legg-Calves Perthes disease; Thyroid disorders

Shiba Inus   Patella luxation; Short spine

Tibetan Spaniels   Medial patella luxation

Tibetan Terriers   Thyroid disorders

HERDING DOGS

Australian Cattle Dogs   OCD of the hock

Australian Shepherds   Hip dysplasia; Dwarfism; Spina bifida

Bearded Collies   Hip dysplasia

Belgian Malinois   Hip dysplasia

Belgian Sheepdogs   Hip dysplasia; Neoplasias

Belgian Tervurens   Hip dysplasia; Thyroid disorders

Border Collies   OCD; Hip dysplasia

Bouviers des Flandres   Elbow dysplasia; Hip dysplasia

Briards   Thyroid disorders; Hip dysplasia

Cardigan Welsh Corgis   Medial patella luxation

Collies (Rough and Smooth)   Dwarfism; Neoplasias

German Shepherd Dogs   Dwarfism; Panosteitis, shown as limb pain and intermittent lameness between the ages of 6 and 12 months; Hip dysplasia; UAP; Cartilagenous Exostosis; Pannus; Elbow dysplasia; Neoplasias; Thyroid disorders; OCD; Degenerative myelopathy causes progressive hind limb paralysis in middle age to older dogs

Old English Sheepdogs   Hip dysplasia; Wobblers syndrome

Pembroke Welsh Corgis   IVD; Hip dysplasia; Swimmers syndrome

Puliks   Hip dysplasia

Shetland Sheepdogs   Hip dysplasia; Dwarfism; Thyroid disorders; Neoplasias; Muscular dystrophy

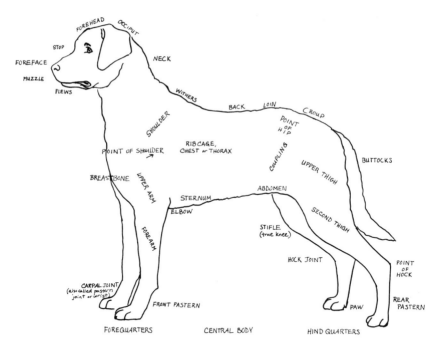

FOREHEAD
OCCIPUT
STOP
FOREFACE
NECK
MUZZLE
FLEWS
WITHERS
BACK
LOIN
CROUP
SHOULDER
POINT OF HIP
RIBCAGE, CHEST or THORAX
POINT OF SHOULDER
COUPLING
UPPER THIGH
BUTTOCKS
BREASTBONE
UPPER ARM
ABDOMEN
STERNUM
ELBOW
SECOND THIGH
FOREARM
STIFLE (true knee)
HOCK JOINT
POINT OF HOCK
CARPAL JOINT (also called pastern joint or wrist)
FRONT PASTERN
PAW
REAR PASTERN
FOREQUARTERS
CENTRAL BODY
HIND QUARTERS

Illustration by Monique Raymond

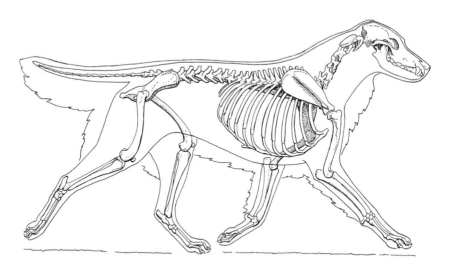

A dog's ability to move in a prescribed manner is dependent upon anatomical structure to support the undertaken activity. Bone, muscle, ligament, and cartilage surface work together to allow the dog to move. The efficiency of the movement is dependent upon proper alignment and the condition of each element.

Illustration by Marcia Schlehr

CHAPTER 3

CANINE ANATOMY AND STRUCTURE

Is your dog structurally sound? Why does it matter?

A dog's ability to move in a prescribed manner depends on anatomical structure to support the activity. Observe a dog in movement. The acts we take for granted: walking, trotting, and running, all result from the combined efforts of various body parts. Bones, muscles, ligaments, and other soft tissues work together to propel the dog. A dog in fluid motion displays the strength of bone, neurological control, the proper conditioning of muscle, and the cardiovascular function. When any of the components become diseased or traumatized, function and movement are impaired.

Dogs cannot tell us when they are in pain—at least not verbally. However, dogs tell us a lot about their health by displaying various body postures. A healthy dog will move, stand, sit, and recline differently from a dog in pain. Irregularity in locomotion or lack of symmetry in muscle mass can be the first clues to identifying underlying disease or injury in the dog.

ASSESSING A DOG

Dog owners should develop observation skills to help identify irregularities early. Some observation skills are somewhat intuitive; others require concentration on specific details. Begin assessing your dog by gathering an impression of the overall dog.

What is the dog's general appearance? The nutritional status and visible muscle mass are easily observable. Swelling or shrinking of a body part should be observable. Know what's normal for your dog—any sudden changes in appearance should be quickly reported to your veterinarian.

Carriage of the head and neck tells a lot about the weight distribution between the front and the rear and about a dog's comfort level. At rest, a healthy dog's head is held up, and it may be carried lower or level with the back while running. A dog that lacks flexibility in the neck may be in great pain.

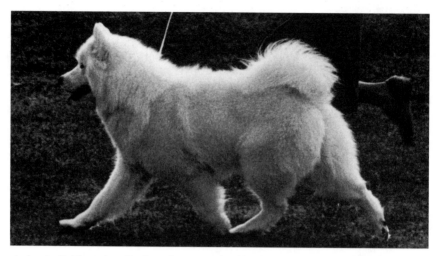

A dog in fluid motion displays the strength of bone, neurological control, the proper conditioning of muscle, and the function of the cardiovascular system.

Photo by Kent and Donna Dannen

Dogs with rear limb problems may carry their head and neck lower than usual. Dogs with front limb problems may carry their head higher. Reluctance to turn the head to the right or left may indicate neck pain associated with intervertebral disk disease or bruising.

Weight distribution while the dog is standing or moving should be even. Shifting weight from a limb, "favoring" a leg, or preferring certain body positions (at rest) may reflect an effort to relieve pain in an isolated area. The space between a moving dog's legs should be consistent in both the front and rear. For example, if a dog moves with its front feet landing four inches apart, the back legs should also show a four-inch width. Breed types vary and the appropriate distance for a particular dog may be defined in the Standard for the given breed. Tracking with unequal widths may indicate orthopedic abnormalities, and dogs exhibiting front or rear widths that are too wide or too narrow should be examined by a veterinarian.

Finally, *tail carriage* also tells us about a dog's comfort level. A relaxed tail carried appropriately for the dog's breed signals good health. A tucked-under tail indicates stress—possibly pain induced.

Disease or injury to any or all body components will cause pain at various levels. Dogs in pain will respond to the degree of discomfort. Dogs with mild discomfort may attempt to continue with routine activity. Dogs moderately affected may exhibit difficulty with stressful activ-

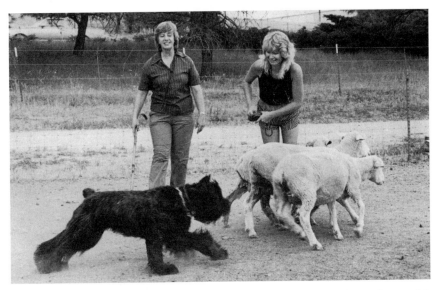

Dogs moderately affected by orthopedic illness may exhibit difficulty with stressful activity, such as getting up and down or running at a moderate pace. This Bouvier des Flandres displays health and vitality in doing the job it was bred to perform.

Photo by Kent and Donna Dannen

ity, such as getting up and down or running at a moderate pace. Dogs in pain will refuse to attempt "normal" actions, will exhibit altered gait, and may display aggression. Dogs thought to be "lazy" may be responding to pain associated with orthopedic unsoundness. Depending on the dog, a dog in any amount of pain may become irritable or aggressive.

Lameness or pain may be the result of injury or disease to any component of the musculoskeletal system. Bone, cartilage, muscle, tendon, ligament, or neurovascular structures can contribute to lameness.

BONES

Bones serve as the supportive and protective framework of the body. They act as levers for the muscles and attach muscles, ligaments, or tendons. Bones support the body structure while maintaining form during movement and locomotion. In order for a dog to perform, it needs healthy bones. When bones are damaged, the dog will experience pain.

Bone is a living substance comprised of fibrous tissue, blood and lymph vessels, nerves, and other substances. Broken bones, or surgi-

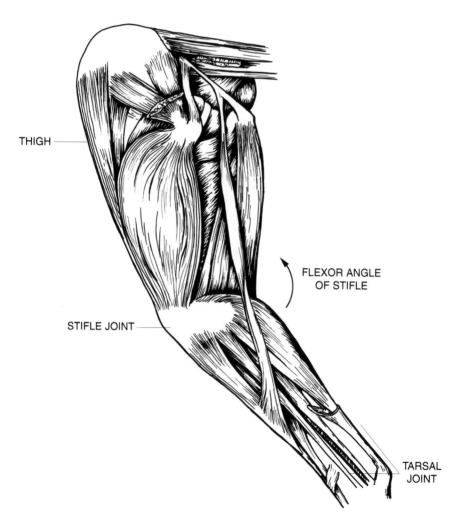

THIGH

FLEXOR ANGLE
OF STIFLE

STIFLE JOINT

TARSAL
JOINT

Anatomy of the rear assembly.   *Illustration by Monique Raymond*

cally altered bones, can heal because bone is capable of remodeling through resorption and reformation.

Modeling (the change of the size, shape, or orientation of bone) occurs during growth and throughout life. The German anatomist Julius Wolff (1836–1902) first observed that a bone can alter its structure to accommodate changes in function. Wolff's law predicts that the thickness of the outer wall (cortex) and the spongy bone in the marrow cavity adapt to the stress placed on the bone.

If the amount of stress increases, the cortex becomes thicker in response to the increased pull or pressure. It does this through the stimulation of new bone production by the outer layer of cells on the cortex (*periosteum*), while the inner layers of cells on the cortex (*endosteum*) are kept from resorbing bone.

Bone is laid down in areas of stress and absorbed in areas of nonstress. Therefore, misaligned bones heal by forming new bone on the compressed or concave side and resorbing the bone on the stretched or convex side. The bone is trying to fill in the perceived defect.

Bone loss occurs when bones are left idle. For example, the space program has studied the effects of weightlessness on bone health of the astronauts. They have discovered that astronauts suffer problems with bone loss/resorption (osteoporosis) from being weightless for extended periods of time. Bones idle from sitting in the space capsule for too long lacked muscle pull, which commonly occurs when performing everyday activities. Physical therapy protocols have been developed to address this concern, and all astronauts exercise in space to provide necessary muscle activity, which prevents bone loss (osteoporosis).

Similar concerns exist for the health of dogs' bones. Dogs that suffer trauma or disease should be treated as soon as possible to prevent bone deterioration. Reduction in function (movement) results in the net loss of bone and can begin within 72 hours of disuse. This occurs with partial or complete paralysis and is also associated with trauma or disease to bones. Repair procedures performed on freshly injured bones often produce good results, but injuries treated after even a few days become more complicated, requiring longer rehabilitation and physical therapy.

Bones are classified according to shape and function. *Long bones* form in the limbs, acting as support columns. Each long bone is composed of a central shaft (*diaphysis*) and two ends (*epiphyses*). The *physis* separates the epiphyses and the diaphysis and is the growth plate in animals. *Short bones* serve to diffuse concussion in the limbs; such bones experience pounding force when a dog runs or lands from a jump. Short bones are found in the wrist (carpus) and ankle (tarsus). *Irregularly shaped bones* form the vertebral column.

The components of bone include the *matrix, periosteum,* and *marrow*. The matrix is located in the shaft and is composed of compacted calcified substance. The periosteum is a membrane covering the outer surface of the bone. The bone marrow occupies the spongy bone space and is essential in blood cell formation.

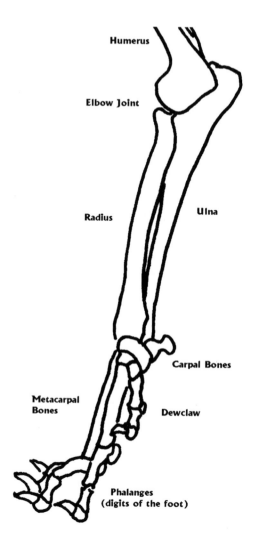

Humerus

Elbow Joint

Radius

Ulna

Carpal Bones

Metacarpal Bones

Dewclaw

Phalanges (digits of the foot)

Bone structure of front limb.

JOINT STRUCTURE

The *scapula* and *humerus* combine to form the shoulder joint. This *ball and socket* joint is capable of movement in any direction, but usually functions in flexion and extension. The distal (or far) end of the humerus joins with the *radius* and *ulna* to form the elbow, a *hinged* joint. The carpal joint (wrist) is located distally to the radius and ulna and consists of several small bones as well as soft tissue structures.

The wrist area is subject to many orthopedic problems for dogs who compete in sporting events (due to the constant strain from jumping and landing on forelimbs). The *metacarpal* (hand) bones are long bones that have a miniaturized appearance. The *phalanges* (fingers or toes) are the bones that make up the digits of the foot.

The *femur* is the largest bone found in the canine skeleton. The close (proximal) end unites with the *pelvic girdle* to form the ball and socket hip joint. The femur joins at the far end (distally) with the *tibia* and *fibula* at the *stifle* (knee) joint. At the far end of the tibia and fibula are the *tarsal* bones that form the hock (ankle), which includes the related soft tissues.

The *metatarsal* bones resemble the metacarpal bones. The *phalanges* of the rear foot are similar to those of the front foot. The first digit, the *dewclaw*, is frequently absent or may vary from a fully developed "toe" to only a vestige of the structure.

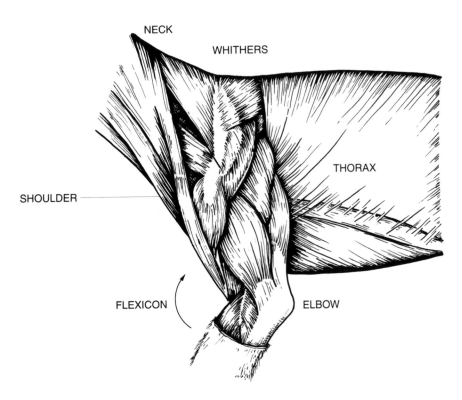

Shoulder and front assembly.   *Illustration by Monique Raymond*

A well-formed joint allows the bones to act as effective levers, and the correct meeting of bones and structures is critical to proper function and range of motion. The *synovial* joint includes the *joint capsule, cavity, joint cartilage,* and *synovial fluid.* The ligaments, fat pads, and each meniscus (crescent-shaped structures) found in the joints and surrounding areas all influence joint structures. The range of motion the joint has is limited by muscles, ligaments, the joint capsule, and the shapes of the bones involved.

Lubrication is vital to a healthy joint. Each joint's type of movement, its workload, and the properties of the synovial fluid all have a

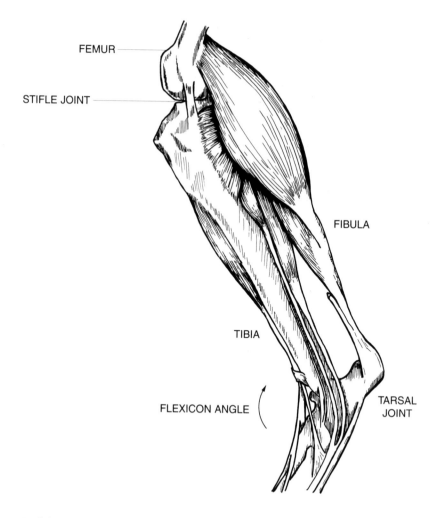

Back leg.   *Illustration by Monique Raymond*

bearing on joint lubrication. It is important to realize that the general health and condition of the dog has a marked influence on the amount of synovial fluid present in the joint.

The *synovial joint membrane* is the highly vascular lining of the joint capsule. This membrane covers all structures within the joint, with the exception of the surface that is in contact with the other side of the joint (articular surface) that is covered by articular cartilage. The synovial cells of the membrane produce the synovial fluid and destroy invading bacteria or other foreign particles.

Articular cartilage gives joints a gliding action and provides resilience. This cartilage lacks blood vessels and nerve endings. It receives nutrition from the synovial fluid. Because of its lack of blood vessels, articular cartilage that has experienced *surface* injury is unable to heal completely. Full thickness injury, however, can heal with help from the underlying bone. Articular cartilage is composed of chondrocytes, fibers, and a matrix consisting of water, collagen, and proteoglycan.

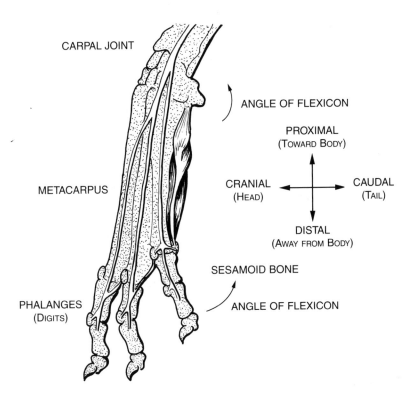

Lateral view of the front paw.   *Illustration by Monique Raymond*

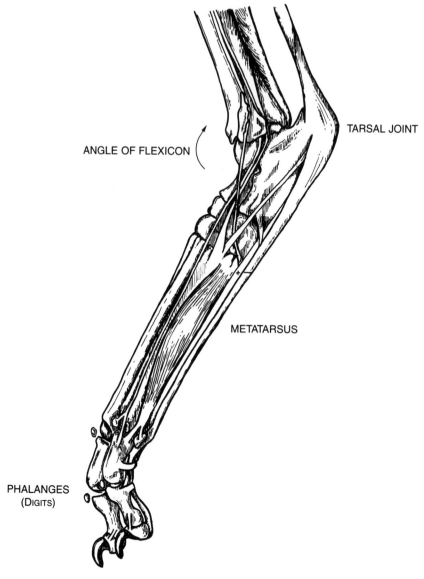

ANGLE OF FLEXICON

TARSAL JOINT

METATARSUS

PHALANGES
(DIGITS)

Right rear tarsus.   *Illustration by Monique Raymond*

Although articular cartilage does not have nerve endings, joint pain is very real and is caused by nerve endings in the joint capsule. Trauma or disease causes an increase in joint fluid, stretching of the joint capsule, and therefore pain.

MUSCULATURE

Muscles provide the necessary power for almost all body functions: locomotion, respiration, circulation, etc. Muscles are classified in three groups: *skeletal muscle, smooth muscle,* and *cardiac muscle.* Skeletal muscle is the voluntary muscle of concern to orthopedics. Smooth muscle is the involuntary muscle in vessels, glands, and organs. Cardiac muscle is the muscle of the heart.

Skeletal muscle consists of fiber bundles, connects to bone by tendons, and comprises approximately one-third to one-half of dogs' total

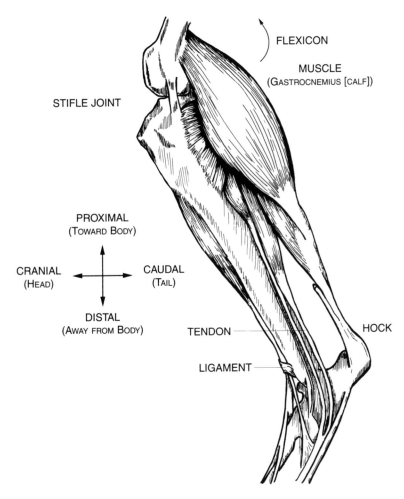

Medial aspect of the stifle.   *Illustration by Monique Raymond*

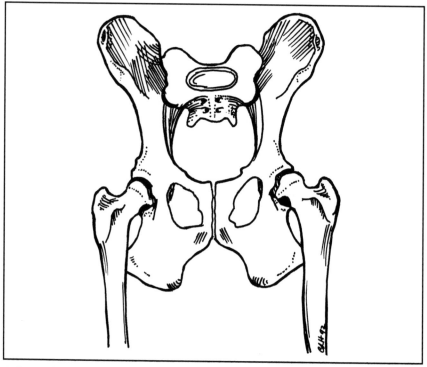

Pelvis and hip joint.

body weight. Understanding the normal anatomic function of muscles is important for effective therapeutic planning.

Some muscles have more than one function, depending on their origin and point of insertion. *Abductors* draw the limb away from the midline of the body, whereas *adductors* pull the limb centrally. *Extensors* straighten limbs, while *flexors* bend or draw the jointed parts together.

Tendons consist of long, regularly arranged connective tissue. They connect muscle to bone and transmit the biomechanical forces developed by the muscles. Tendons can act like a modified pulley to alter their direction over a joint. The elasticity of the tendon may reduce a sudden force acting on a muscle, thereby preventing injury to the muscle. Tendon injury is often related to trauma when overwhelming force has been applied to the muscle tendon unit.

Ligaments consist of dense connective tissue. They connect bones to other bones, providing stability to joints while guiding motion within the

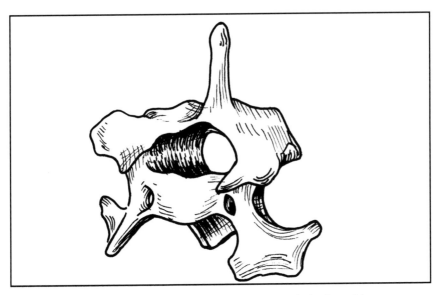

The vertebral column consists of approximately 50 irregularly shaped bones, or vertebrae like this one.   *Illustration by Monique Raymond*

joint. Ligaments are responsible for supplying information through nerve fibers regarding the position of the limbs. Ligaments are less elastic than tendons, and their tendency to become damaged increases with maturity of the dog. Younger pets, like young children, are more predisposed to fractures than to ligament ruptures; older pets may develop ligament ruptures rather than bone fractures.

SPINAL STRUCTURE

The vertebral column consists of approximately 50 irregularly shaped bones. The classification of the vertebral column is arranged based on location from *cervical* (neck), *thoracic* (chest), *lumbar* (lower back), *sacral* (hip) and *coccygeal* (tail). The vertebral column flexes and extends as well as functions in the locomotion of the body. A healthy spine and support structures are critical to keeping a dog functional.

The first letter of the word naming the specific area (such as "C" for cervical), coupled with the number of the vertebrae in that area, constitutes the vertebral formula. Dogs are C_7, T_{13}, L_7, S_3, and Cy_{20+}. (The number 20 is arbitrary for the coccygeal vertebrae; many dogs have fewer and a few have more.) In other words, C_5 stands for the fifth cervical vertebra.

Although the amount of movement between any two vertebrae is limited, the vertebral column is quite flexible. The three sacral vertebrae, which do not have disks, fuse to form the sacrum. All other vertebrae remain separate and articulate with contiguous vertebrae in forming movable, disk-lined joints.

Meninges, membranes that cover the spinal cord, protect the spinal cord from injury.

CHAPTER 4

CASE REPORTS

Rebecca came to the animal hospital in tears. She had brought her Golden Retriever 70 miles for a consultation because her veterinarian had diagnosed hip dysplasia. Rebecca was distraught; she loved this dog and didn't want to lose her. Rebecca knew that Diamond had a serious disease; what she didn't know was that the effects of the disease were fixable.

Diagnosis of orthopedic disease often puts dog owners into a state of shock. Although a veterinarian may have explained the technical implications of the problem, many times the emotional implications are overlooked. A diagnosis of hip dysplasia, a torn cruciate ligament, or intervertebral disk disease (IVD) is certainly not a welcome event, but each of these conditions is potentially correctable.

What happens after crippling disease has been diagnosed in the dog? Identification of treatment options and selection of the treatment route follows the diagnosis. Bad news and good news awaits the owners of otherwise healthy dogs that are affected by joint, neurological, and many other diseases:

The bad news: Some orthopedic (and related) diseases respond to conservative treatment, but many require reconstructive surgery to return the dog to an active lifestyle.

The good news: Technology has advanced so far that most orthopedic surgeries have excellent prognoses for dogs to fully recover. Surgical specialists practice across the country, making the surgeries accessible to most people.

Rebecca listened carefully to the doctor as he explained that Diamond's hip dysplasia was quite severe. And she shed tears of joy hearing that total hip replacement was a very successful procedure and that Diamond was a great candidate for the surgery. Diamond's left hip was replaced a few weeks later. The right hip was replaced a few months later. Both dog and owner are doing fine.

Rebecca's story is typical of many dog owners. We like happy endings, and most orthopedic cases have similar outcomes.

BAXTER

Before a young couple left for vacation last August, they made arrangements to board their dog, Baxter, at a local kennel. Little did they know that the brief kennel stay would uncover a congenital problem in the dog that would require major surgery.

After the couple left Baxter at the boarding kennel, the dog enjoyed the environment, expressing his exuberance by barking, jumping, and frolicking in the kennel run. The activity took its toll, however, and kennel personnel noticed that the dog began to limp. Eventually Baxter experienced difficulty standing up and lying down. Thinking the dog had injured himself, kennel personnel took Baxter to a local veterinarian. After examination and review of the dog's hip x-rays, dysplasia was suspected. This genetic defect was unmasked by the dog's unusual activity level. However, even with normal activity, the symptoms would have eventually become apparent.

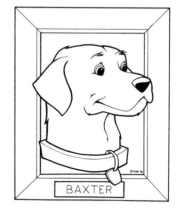

Baxter, a Labrador Retriever, suffered from canine hip dysplasia.

Illustration by Stone Perelas

Baxter was referred to an orthopedic specialist for further examination. The dog's owners soon discovered that the kennel stay and the associated veterinary involvement were a blessing in disguise. Baxter's condition was at a point that left surgical options open that upon further deterioration of the hip joint would have been unavailable.

Baxter's examination began with observation of the dog's gait and standing postures. When the movement raised questions about soundness, Baxter was anesthetized and his hip joints were palpated. X-rays confirmed suspicions, and surgery was recommended to correct Baxter's orthopedic problems.

Because Baxter's dysplasia was caught early, he was a good candidate for a procedure known as triple pelvic osteotomy. The surgery was performed within a week of the diagnosis, and Baxter began his road to recovery. Following surgery, Baxter stayed at the hospital for five days. After Baxter's release, his owners were instructed to confine him to a crate to keep him quiet, and they were provided with an Elizabethan collar to keep the dog from chewing the sutures. Walks were limited to those needed for elimination, and slippery surfaces were avoided.

Today Baxter leads a full life with no limitations on activity. One of his owners, Susan, describes him as a typical Lab. He enjoys running through the hills, and he loves to romp with his pal Molly, a Golden Retriever.

MUFFIN

Muffin, a three-year-old Lhasa Apso, was referred to an animal behaviorist/trainer, Diane, for a consultation regarding the dog's aggression toward people. The dog had been growling, was reluctant to be handled, and had bitten her family members, the Bakers. The dog had never been abused or reprimanded with harsh physical punishments. What was causing Muffin's aggression?

In order to examine the dog, the owners presented her to the behaviorist by handing her backward to Diane (teeth facing away from her). After intro-ductory measures, the behaviorist was

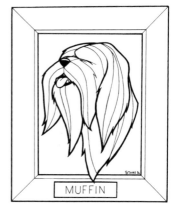

Luxating patellas were found in Muffin, a Lhasa Apso.
Illustration by Stone Perelas

able to perform a standard behavior analysis. By lying the dog on her side, Diane evaluated handlability and dominant/submissive tendencies. While stroking the dog she noticed something quite unexpected—she felt the knee pop in and out. Could pain be responsible for Muffin's ill temper?

Diane knew that subluxating patellas were common in Lhasa Apsos. She suggested that the Bakers have Muffin evaluated by a veterinarian to assess the health of the knee joints. The Bakers complied, and the physical examination confirmed Diane's suspicions. The dog was referred to an orthopedic specialist, the knee was repaired, and the dog has fully healed from the surgery.

The Bakers report a significant change in Muffin's demeanor, which is attributed to pain relief associated with the surgery. However, Muffin and her family are still addressing her dominance/aggressive tendencies. Now that the knee has been fixed, Muffin is ready for an attitude adjustment.

FOXIE

Foxie the Dachsie (Dachshund) leads a "dog's life." She is the treasured companion of Tom and Eloise, whose children have grown and left home. Foxie fills a need for her owners, people who enjoy nurturing and who think of Foxie as their surrogate child and give her all the creature comforts. She is Eloise's constant companion, is well fed, visits the veterinarian and the groomer regularly, and shares her owners' bed—until recently.

Shortly after Foxie turned two years old she paid a price for her "lifestyle." The beloved little dog was going about her daily rituals and jumped up onto the bed to watch Eloise get ready to go out. However, this day was not like the others. As Foxie jumped she let out a loud cry, and she wasn't able to get up.

Eloise, though panicked at the sight of the injured Foxie, kept her cool. She called the veterinarian, who explained that the situation was not that unusual.

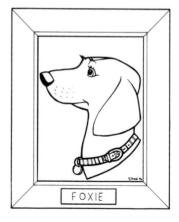

FOXIE

Typical of many in her breed, Foxie the Dachsie (Dachshund) ruptured a disk in her spine.
Illustration by Stone Perelas

Dachshunds (because of the proportion of their backs to their leg lengths and because of their abnormal disks) often suffer spinal cord damage. The doctor advised Eloise to take her dog to a specialty clinic for assessment, knowing that the dog was in pain and probably needed disk surgery. The orthopedic veterinarian explained that Foxie's abnormal disks would have eventually ruptured with even slight stress, such as stepping off a curb.

Diagnostic tests were ordered, and the myelogram showed the disk compressing the cord and that other disks in the area had calcified and could present problems in the future. The surgeon explained that Foxie had an excellent prognosis for a full recovery if she underwent surgery right away. During surgery the doctor removed the disk that was pressing on the spinal cord. Then the surgeon removed the calcified disks (via fenestration) that threatened to rupture in the future.

It took Foxie about three months to fully recover, but with time and physical therapy, Foxie is running around as before, but she's not jumping on the bed!

RED

Red, a Doberman, is the perfect height to rest his chin on his owner's lap when David sits in the recliner. This minor characteristic may have saved Red's life. Red developed a disease known as wobblers syndrome, which is common to the breed. Because of the head-resting habit, David noticed that Red had stopped picking up his head to place it on David's lap because the dog's neck hurt. David missed this bonding ritual and noticed the dog's reluctance to participate in a formerly enjoyable act. He watched closely and realized Red didn't turn his head when called. Red seemed a little unsure of himself and seemed a little wobbly when he walked.

David knew something was wrong, so he took Red to his veterinarian for a checkup. Wobblers syndrome was diagnosed early, allowing it to be treated successfully. The veterinarian started with conservative treatment, prescribing a drug used to relieve pain and inflammation (prednisone) and plenty of rest for the dog. This helped, but David became concerned about Red's long-term health, and he researched the disease by calling Red's breeder. The breeder was quite familiar with the disease, but she was surprised that Red was affected. She had carefully screened Red's parents, and neither had a history of wobblers syndrome in their pedigree. The breeder advised David that wobblers syndrome is common in Dobermans and, if left untreated for very long, can carry a worse prognosis and be harder to treat. She also advised David to seek a second opinion, and she recommended a surgeon at a referral practice.

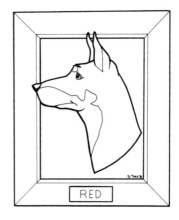

Red, a noble Doberman, "wobbled" when walking, consistent with cervical instability.
Illustration by Stone Perelas

The diagnosis of cervical vertebral instability (wobblers syndrome) was confirmed by the specialist, and he presented David with all the treatment options and prognoses. His recommended treatment was surgery. Today Red is once again enjoying his evenings with his head on David's lap.

SAMMY

Keeping in good physical condition is the goal of many, and an exercise routine is part of the plan. John knew the importance of keeping fit, and he thought that running with his dog would keep Sammy healthy. One day when John and Sammy crossed a railroad track bridge, Sammy watched as John fell down the ravine before the bridge. Then, instead of going back and forth down the ravine, Sammy, who was trained to stay with his owner, jumped

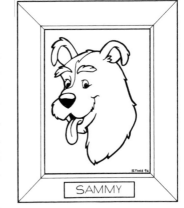

Sammy, a mixed-breed dog, jumped and injured his carpi.
Illustration by Stone Perelas

from the bridge to stay with John. Although it was only about 10 feet down from where Sammy jumped, the force of the landing caused both carpal joints (wrists) to hyperextend and slip out of place, tearing the ligaments. No bones were broken, but he couldn't use his front legs. John luckily suffered no injury, so he carried Sammy home and brought him to the veterinarian immediately.

Because of the severity of the injuries and the complete dislocation suffered, reconstruction with ligament repair was not appropriate (a subluxated carpal joint can be reconstructed, but a fully luxated carpus requires more extensive surgery). Fusion of the joint became the procedure of choice. The veterinarian had seen cases like Sammy's before because severe carpal or tarsal sprains are common. This fusion (arthrodesis) is performed more often in the carpus than in any other joint, because such injuries to the carpus and tarsus respond poorly to other treatments and limb function is not adversely affected by arthrodesis of these joints (arthrodesis of all other joints will dramatically change limb function).

Surgery was performed on both legs at the same time because Sammy couldn't use either one. After surgery Sammy wore splints for four months, but at least he could walk during that time. Today Sammy enjoys a full life. John still takes Sammy jogging with him, but they don't go to the railroad track bridge anymore, and they take it a little slower.

BARON

Baron's shoulders required surgery to remove OCD (osteochondritis dissecans) lesions on both sides. Today Baron is pain free and very active, but he experienced pain for about three months during puppyhood before a definitive diagnosis was made and surgery performed.

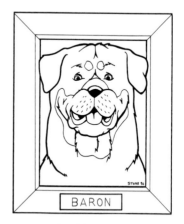

Looking back, his owners realized that Baron first started limping after a day of playing with a neighbor's dog. The dogs enjoyed roughhousing, and Baron's owners thought that he was just sore from too much exercising. When Baron seemed to improve, Frank and Susan assumed that their conclusion was right. But within a few weeks, they realized Baron was still limping on the same front leg, just not as badly. They brought Baron to their veterinarian, who recommended exercise

Baron's shoulders required repair, due to growth related causes typical of a fast-growing Rottweiler.
Illustration by Stone Perelas

restriction and aspirin, but was unable to definitively diagnose the problem.

A month later Frank and Susan returned to the animal hospital because Baron still seemed to be in pain. The veterinarian was able to elicit pain when the right shoulder was extended. X-rays of the right shoulder were taken, which showed an OCD lesion. Because OCD is often bilateral, the other shoulder was x-rayed, which disclosed an OCD lesion there as well.

Baron was given cage confinement for four weeks to see if the clinical signs would regress, as sometimes occurs with OCD. After one month, lameness in the right foreleg remained, so they chose surgical removal of the OCD fragments in both shoulders. Even though Baron wasn't lame on the left foreleg—possibly because he had no choice but to use the "best of the worst" of his legs—the OCD lesion was removed. Had surgery on the left leg been delayed, once the right shoulder was fixed and no longer hurting, the left shoulder would then probably have been more painful, and lameness would occur. Baron would have to undergo two surgeries and recovery periods instead of one.

WINDY

Windy is a beautiful Border Collie. She loves to run and jump, so when she became a champion fly ball catcher, no one was surprised, least of all her people, Sam and Donna. But Donna was surprised when Sam and Windy came home from a tournament, not only without a ribbon, but with Windy not using one of her back legs. Sam and Donna thought Windy was in great shape and so strong that nothing could ever hurt her.

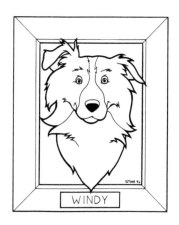

Windy, a Border Collie, tore a ligament in her knee while attempting to catch a ball.
Illustration by Stone Perelas

They took Windy to see their veterinarian right away, and he diagnosed a ruptured anterior cruciate ligament (RACL). The veterinarian knew Windy was a young athlete with a lot of years ahead of her, and if she were to continue to compete (or even enjoy running and jumping), she would need to have the knee fixed correctly and right away, before degenerative changes occurred.

Windy underwent surgery to repair her knee and was kept very quiet for four weeks afterward. The second month after surgery she started taking short walks, gradually building up distance. Today she is back catching balls and jumping hurdles, and she's still one of the best.

Sam and Donna now know that Windy was a perfect candidate for a RACL because she is so well-muscled and jumps and turns a lot. They are watching her closely for signs of problems in the other knee, so if she gets hurt they can fix it right away and prevent long-term problems.

MONSTER

Not all knee injuries are as obvious as a dog that cannot use a leg at all.

Monster was the sweetest American Pit Bull Terrier you ever met. The neighborhood kids nicknamed him the "Good Monster" of the block. Monster was very strong, and the kids liked him to pull them around in a wagon. Monster (and his owner Jill) would always comply of course, but every now and then Monster showed some reluctance. He would limp, and his right hind leg hurt.

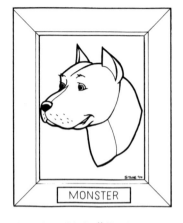

MONSTER

American Pit Bull Terrier, Monster, suffered a slow and progressive tearing of the cruciate ligament in his knee.
Illustration by Stone Perelas

Jill brought him to the veterinarian a few times for evaluation, and although Monster's knee obviously was hurting, the doctor couldn't find anything wrong with the joint. Usually after a few days of rest and aspirin, Monster would feel better. After a while though, the episodes of pain and limping seemed to last longer and happen more often. Although Monster remained happy and good-natured, it was now obvious that something was bothering him. Jill took him to a specialist who watched Monster walk in different directions and in circles. The veterinarian felt the dog all over, and when the exam was done, the doctor suspected that Monster had torn (either partially or completely) a cruciate ligament in his knee over the last few weeks. But because Monster was so strong, the vet couldn't tell for sure since Monster's muscles held the knee so tightly that the vet couldn't manipulate it well. To get around the muscle-tightening dilemma, the veterinarian sedated Monster and palpated the knee with the dog fully relaxed. Sure enough, the knee moved forward and back in an uncharacteristic manner. An x-ray showed arthritis starting to form because of the abnormal movement in the damaged knee and the recurrence of the injury. A torn cruciate ligament was found to be the cause. Surgery was performed on the dog, and today, although Monster now has a little arthritis in that knee, he leads a happy, active life.

BUCK, SALLY, AND DAISY

Jennifer loves dogs. She teaches Obedience classes and puppy kindergarten classes on Wednesdays and Saturdays. Jennifer's students learn more about dog care than just how to teach them to Sit and to Come. She shares information on flea control and grooming, and she stresses the importance of maintaining a health program and visiting the veterinarian regularly.

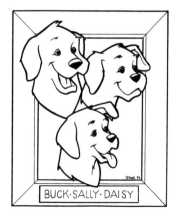

BUCK·SALLY·DAISY

Elbow dysplasia kept Buck, Sally, and Daisy, Golden Retriever puppies, from walking.
Illustration by Stone Perelas

Jennifer enjoys the recommendations of many people in the dog community. One breeder sent her some puppies to train as a group. These Golden Retriever puppies had great temperaments and learned quickly. One week, when the puppies were about four and one-half months old, Jennifer received a call from Buck's owner, reporting that her puppy was whining and didn't like to go for walks anymore. Jennifer told the caller to take Buck for a checkup, which resulted in a diagnosis of elbow dysplasia. Buck underwent corrective surgery to repair the joint, which promised to return him to full function.

A week after the call from Buck's owner, Sally's owner reported similar symptoms. Then Daisy's owner noticed that her dog slowed down, eventually refusing to get up. Both of Buck's littermates were diagnosed and treated for elbow dysplasia, and Daisy also had hip dysplasia on the left side. The dogs were surgically corrected and today lead normal lives, but the appearance of the disease in several puppies in the litter underscores the genetic influence.

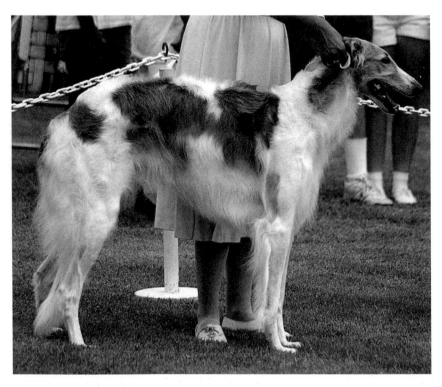

If you take a proactive approach to your dog's well-being, you can position your-self to identify strengths and weaknesses and develop a game plan to fit your dog's needs. Good breeding, good nutrition, and good exercise help keep dogs in peak condition, like this Borzoi.

CHAPTER 5

LAMENESS DIAGNOSIS

Why look for problems in your dog? Early diagnosis of orthopedic problems allows for early treatment, minimizing discomfort and preventing further progression of the problem. Furthermore, it identifies problems in potential breeding stock prior to using those who will prove to be affected. Lameness is often the first observable symptom of orthopedic problems in dogs.

Often a pet owner will notice an awkward gait or pain associated with movement, which signals that a veterinary examination is in order. By the time the symptoms are noticed, however, the pet and the owner may have lost valuable time in treating the cause of the problem.

As a dog owner, you are the first line of the offense. If you take a proactive approach to your dog's well-being, you can position yourself to identify strengths and weaknesses and develop a game plan to fit your dog's needs.

Begin by acquainting yourself with the diseases that threaten your dog's breed or type and regularly study your dog's movement. Discuss these concerns with your veterinarian, trainer, and breeder, and seek help as soon as you notice an irregularity.

An irregular gait, the exhibition of pain during movement, or the failure to utilize a limb can be described as lameness. While some lameness is crippling, other types are barely detectable. Lameness should *always* be taken seriously, regardless of severity.

Dog owners can provide needed help in assessing dogs' soundness. Dogs should be watched for subtle signs that preclude the development of lameness. This is especially important with growing dogs and large dogs. Regular examinations should be performed by the veterinarian and the owner to ensure that their dogs' orthopedic soundness is not diminished.

Decreased range of motion is often the first symptom of joint problems observed. Dogs with joint swelling or capsular scarring (due to poor joint conformation) will suffer. When these conditions occur, the dog's range of motion is diminished. A dog with limited range of motion will not display proper reach (the outward extension of the

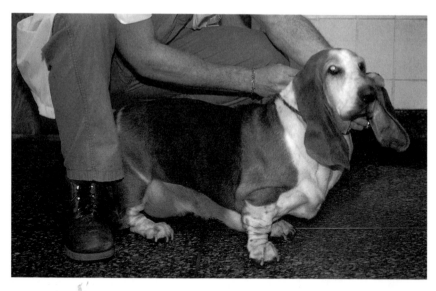

Lameness is often the first observed symptom of orthopedic problems in dogs. The owner of this Basset Hound noticed an awkward gait and pain associated with movement, which signaled that a veterinary examination was in order.

front legs while moving at a trot) and drive (the backward extension of the rear legs while moving at a trot). This limited extension can be the first sign of underlying structural problems.

Whenever range of motion does not seem normal, or when dogs display differences in motion between their right and left sides, suspect pain. Observe the dog at rest and in motion. Palpate the hips and elbows; schedule a veterinary consultation and confirm suspicions with x-rays. Don't hesitate to acquire second opinions or to consult with a veterinary orthopedic specialist.

ASSESSING SOUNDNESS

Observation, gait analysis, and palpation techniques allow veterinarians and trained dog owners to periodically assess dogs' orthopedic soundness. Assessment provides opportunities to recognize problems in the early stages and to provide appropriate treatment, minimizing pain and suffering for the dog.

Why look for trouble? Early diagnosis of structural deficiencies provides treatment options that may not exist later if a condition is left to progress unnoticed. Chances for a return to full function are greatly improved when problems are detected and treated early.

Learn to examine your dog and quickly report any unusual findings to your veterinarian. Under a watchful (or trained) eye, something as subtle as decreased range of motion (extent of movement) of the pelvic limbs can be the first observed symptom of an orthopedic disease such as hip dysplasia. Loss of range of motion can be detected even before lameness arises, which can provide opportunities for early treatment. As lameness progresses, eventually the animal can no longer stand the discomfort, and the lameness will become apparent even to the *un*trained eye. But by this point, degeneration is usually extensive, eliminating some treatment options. Early diagnosis is preferable for all involved: veterinarian, dog owner, and *especially* the dog.

RECOGNIZING LAMENESS

Lameness causes shortened stride and, as we have said, decreased range of motion. Lameness in dogs can be caused by joint effusions, adhesions, trauma, infection, muscle incompetence, or neurological deficit. If left untreated, unequal weight bearing on the limbs may produce further orthopedic problems. For example, hip dysplasia left untreated can predispose a dog to development of anterior cruciate ligament rupture. A dysplastic dog with limited hip joint range of motion will rely upon hyperextension of the knee to lengthen stride and compensate for improper hip function.

Some outward signs of lameness are the following:

- Altered gait

- Favored leg

- Shortened stride

- Increased or decreased range of joint motion

- Abduction or adduction of a limb

- Head-bob associated with placing weight on the affected limb

- Weight carried abnormally in the front or rear

- Stance change (wider or narrower than normal)

OBSERVATION

Observe your dog in a normal standing position. Look for symmetry, balance, and expected conformation *for the breed*. A Dachshund's conformation will vary greatly from that of a Labrador Retriever. Each breed's Standard will specify what is correct for that breed.

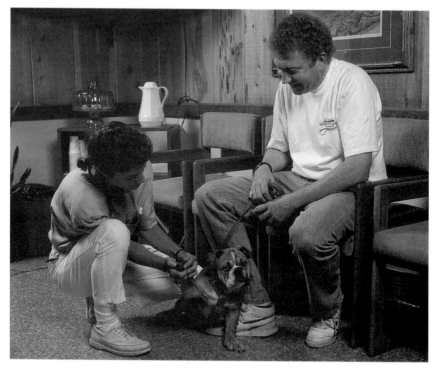

Discuss concerns with your dog's veterinarian, trainer, and breeder, and seek help as soon as you notice an irregularity. Dr. Suzy Lee discusses orthopedic soundness here with a Bulldog owner during a routine puppy exam

At this stage, allow the dog to move and stand naturally. Don't stack the dog or try to influence movement. Note any unusual postures or behaviors. Reluctance to stand may indicate muscle weakness or pain. Straightness of the back and weight transfer from the front to the rear can indicate elbow dysplasia. Broken nails or splayed and hyperextended toe joints may indicate a ligament rupture, an autoimmune problem, or a neurological dysfunction.

GAIT ANALYSIS

Use your keen observation skills to analyze your dog's gait. This analysis may reveal lameness that previously went undetected. Take the time to examine each of your dogs, *even if you don't suspect orthopedic problems.*

Each test requires a dog handler and an observer (usually the veterinarian or a trained individual). To be effective, the exercises must be performed on flat, well-lighted, non-skid surfaces. Use a short leash to best control the dog's movement, and work in an area that presents few distractions for the dog.

The analysis consists of six simple exercises, which will show a variety of angles for observing the dog. Perform the exercises in the order presented here, but if lameness is readily apparent after performing the first two exercises, discontinue the series of tests. If the dog is experiencing lameness, it is also feeling pain. Once lameness is identified, there is no reason to continue to bring pain to the dog.

Exercise 1: Walk/Trot in a Straight Line

As the observer watches, the dog is led straight away and back. This pattern is repeated several times, first with the dog moving at a slow speed and then at a trot. The observer should stand normally and, from time to time during the test, should squat with knees bent while taking note of the following:

- Assess the angle of the patient's head carriage to see if weight is being transferred from the front legs to the back or vice versa. Most quadrupeds carry 60% of their weight on the forelegs and 40% on the rear. Raising or lowering the head may change the fulcrum point of the foreleg muscle group, allowing weight to transfer away from or toward the rear limbs.

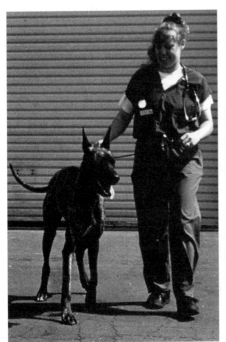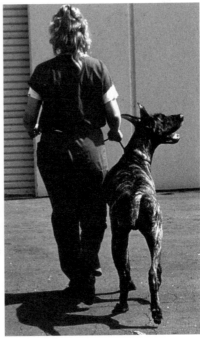

As the observer watches, the dog is led straight away and back. This procedure is repeated several times with the dog moving at a slow speed and then at a trot.

- Observe the patient walking and stopping. Assess any recurrent transfer of weight on the upper section of the leg, close to the patient's center of gravity. One leg left out in front or tucked behind the body may indicate that the dog is experiencing pain.

Exercise 2: Walk in a Circle

The handler should move the dog in a circle with the observer approximately 10 feet away in the center of the circle. Move the dog first clockwise, then counterclockwise.

Circling the dog *toward* an affected limb causes increased weight bearing on the inner leg and may intensify lameness. Look for lameness, muscle atrophy, and weakness on each side, front and rear. Use a slow pace, maintaining a constant, slow speed throughout the exercise. Fast gaits can hide subtle lameness.

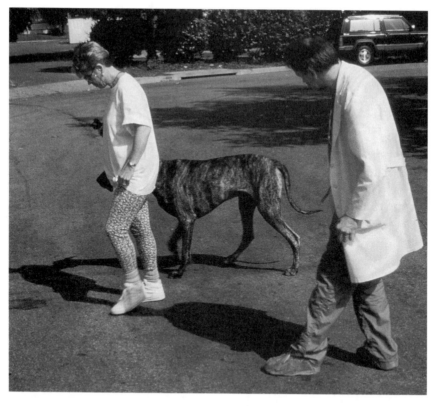

Circling the dog toward an affected limb causes increased weight bearing on the inner leg and may intensify lameness.

Exercise 3: Walk in a Figure 8

Walk your dog through a figure-8 pattern. Change speed occasionally as you complete several executions of the figure 8. Perform the exercise in both directions. When smaller circles are performed, the intensity of lameness may increase, allowing easy recognition of weaknesses in gait.

Assess foot placement and neurological competence as the dog walks in small circles. Nail dragging or stumbling may indicate neurological dysfunction.

If a dog completes the first three exercises without showing signs of lameness, continue to test its soundness. Proceed to exercises four through six, which are more challenging.

Exercise 4: Obstacle Course

Run the patient through an obstacle course consisting of items that test coordination, jumping agility, left and right turns, and stopping. Assess the dog for weakness, lameness, or avoidance of an activity. For example, if during a jump or start of a run, the dog hops or tucks both rear legs under at the same time, the dog may be suffering from orthopedically induced pain. This may indicate weakness in one or both rear legs. Do not force a jump; it could produce pain or further injury.

Exercise 5: Sand or Mud Puddle Test

Walking a dog through sand or a mud puddle allows further assessment of stride symmetry and length. It uncovers unequal weight transfer from limb to limb, which indicates orthopedic problems. After the dog is walked through the selected medium, return to examine the tracks. Measure the depth of the footprints and the distance between prints. Is the dog favoring one side over the other? The footprints will illustrate such differences.

Exercise 6: Painted Toenails

When neurological problems are suspected but not displayed during gait analysis, try this test. Put polish on the dog's nails, both front and rear. Allow the dog 24 hours of normal activity at home. At the end of the test period, examine the wear. Is the wear evenly distributed? If not, suspect neurological dysfunction.

The top of the nails should show no wear, nor should the sides. Uneven wear may indicate a problem associated with dragging the feet. Diagnostic tests including x-rays, myelograms, CT scans, or MRI films may be ordered to help identify the specific disease process at hand.

PALPATION

Palpation of a dog's joints takes but a few minutes, but can be extremely effective in detecting structural deformities. Palpation techniques are simple, and with adequate training, palpation can be performed as part of a veterinary examination by an animal health technician. Basic techniques are performed without the use of anesthesia, however, *only those who are thoroughly trained in these techniques should attempt palpating for structural abnormalities.*

A trained professional may suspect hip dysplasia in young dogs when using palpation, even when x-rays fail to identify malformations. Proper orthopedic examination followed by radiographs (when indicated) can reveal structural problems in time to correct them before further joint degeneration occurs.

Throughout the procedure, keep the dog as comfortable as possible. Allow the dog to stand and lean against you for support when necessary. Be sure to assess the dog's temperament prior to performing palpation; do not force palpation on a dog that is vicious or in obvious pain.

BASIC EXAMINATION

After the gait analysis, stand over the pet's mid-back area. Assess each dog for individual symmetry, even within a breed type. Consider the dog systematically, beginning with the feet. Probe gently but firmly, paying close attention to the pet's reaction.

Be cautious if the animal's temperament is questionable or the person holding the dog does not have adequate control to prevent aggressive behavior. Gentle probing of a specific area may bring a mild or sharp pain response, indicating the cause of lameness. Do not pursue a painful area; note it and report it to your veterinarian. Compare each limb to the opposite side, noting abnormalities. Variations in symmetry, however subtle, from side to side could indicate a problem.

A typical orthopedic examination should include each joint and supporting structure. Study your dog's orthopedic condition and consider each of the following.

TOES AND FOOT POSTURE

Look for hair loss, swelling, and abrasions. Check the nails for inconsistent wear. Are the inner nails worn more than the outer ones? Examine the inner foot for split pads, cracks, or redness.

Gradually extend the exam from the foot pad up each toe, feeling for firm or soft swelling. Feel the tendons, ligaments, muscles, and

After the gait analysis, stand over the pet's mid-back area. Assess each dog for individual symmetry, even within a breed type. Hold the dog steady, grasp the dog's chin, and move the head in several directions: up, down, and in circular motions. Take note of any sign of pain.

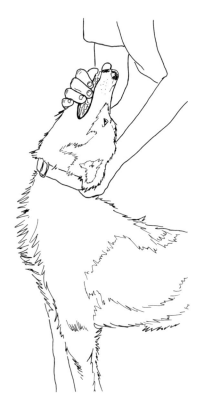

bones for any abnormalities. Check each joint for abnormal range of motion or joint effusion. Pay close attention to possible asymmetry by comparing an abnormal area to the other side.

UPPER MUSCLES OF THE FORELEG

Look for ligament swelling or muscle atrophy. A normal dog will have two finger widths of distance between the point of the shoulder (proximal humerus) and the wrist (radiocarpal articulation) when the elbow is flexed. A width greater than two fingers may indicate elbow dysplasia or other causes of osteoarthrosis of the elbow joint, warranting radiographic assessment.

SHOULDER

Examine (palpate) the scapula, looking for asymmetry and muscle atrophy. Slow flexion of the shoulder joint while gently applying downward pressure on the blade of the scapula and lateral extension of the limb

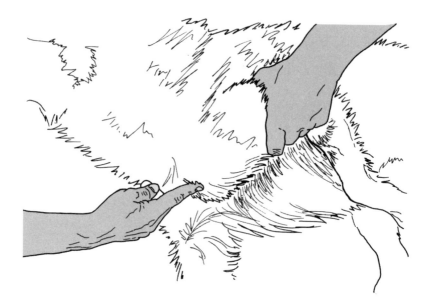

Palpation of the scapula may reveal asymmetry and muscle atrophy in the shoulder. Slow flexion of the shoulder joint while gently applying downward pressure on the blade of the scapula and lateral extension of the limb will allow assessment of the shoulder joint.   *Illustration by Monique Raymond*

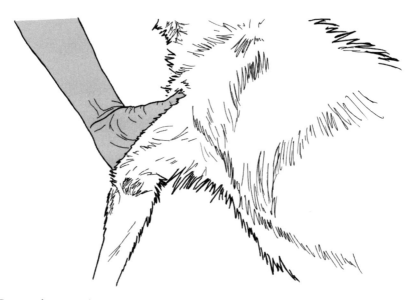

Deep palpation of the muscular joint between the scapula, the humerus, and the thoracic body wall may be indicated in athletic breeds or when previous trauma has occurred in this area.   *Illustration by Monique Raymond*

will allow assessment of the shoulder joint. Pain or reluctance to display a full range of motion may indicate the area is a problem. Comparing the test on the opposite limb may help separate a painful area from the pet's natural resistance to palpation in general.

Deep palpation of the muscular joint between the scapula, the humerus, and the thoracic body wall may be indicated in athletic breeds or when previous trauma has occurred in this area.

PALPATING THE ELBOWS

Elbow dysplasia is one of the most under-diagnosed conditions in dogs and has been found in significant numbers in 36 of 86 breeds evaluated by the Orthopedic Foundation for Animals (OFA). Because this condition is more common than previously thought, veterinarians must pay closer attention to the condition. However, initial screening need not be difficult or costly. Use palpation to assess your dog's elbow joint integrity.

To examine a dog for elbow dysplasia, begin with the two-fingers test. Carefully lift the front leg of the dog off the ground vertically. Gently but firmly push the foreleg up close to the shoulder. Holding your index

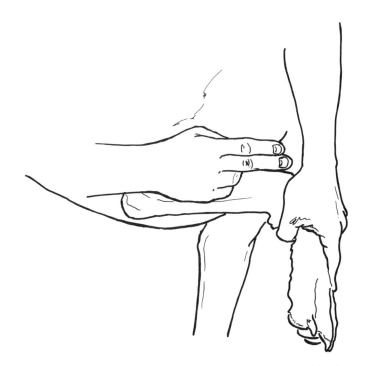

A dog with normal elbow structure will have a distance the width of two fingers between the point of the shoulder (proximal humerus) and the wrist (radiocarpal articulation).   *Illustration by Monique Raymond*

finger and forefinger together, place them between the point of the shoulder and the radial carpal joint as illustrated above. As you conduct the test, allow the dog to lean against you for support.

A dog with normal elbow structure will have a distance the width of two fingers between the point of the shoulder and the wrist. Be certain to ensure that you don't slide your fingers down the angle, or your reading will be inaccurate. A width greater than two fingers indicates decreased range of motion, which may indicate elbow dysplasia or osteoarthrosis of the elbow joint.

PALPATING THE NECK

Holding the dog steady, grasp the dog's chin and move the head in several directions: up, down, and in circular motions. Be careful to avoid a struggle with the dog, and discontinue the exam if the dog fights or pulls away. Signs of pain could indicate disk disease or cervical instability and a need to have the dog examined by a veterinarian.

EXAMINING THE HIPS

Hip dysplasia is an inherited condition. Large breeds are more likely to be affected than small ones. The degeneration that occurs with hip dysplasia is a dynamic process, but the trained and observant dog owner can recognize the condition long before the dog shows symptoms. Early diagnosis provides treatment options that will not exist once the cartilage has degenerated. At that point, the joint becomes severely damaged.

Recently, experts have recognized that hip dysplasia is affected by *the depth of the acetabulum,* (the size of the cup on the pelvis that houses the ball of the femur) and *the degree of joint laxity* (the ease at which the ball of the femur can be popped out of the acetabulum). Radiographs of young dogs' hips may not reflect subtle changes that will become evident later. Some dogs that show adequate cup depth on x-rays develop osteoarthrosis, caused by increased joint laxity. Effective diagnosis of hip dysplasia requires palpation (most beneficial when done by a professional) assessing laxity and radiographs assessing cup depth.

Dysplasia genes become evident as a dog grows, and the influence of exercise and diet can encourage symptoms. Young dogs may not exhibit obvious signs of dysplasia, even though the condition may exist. (Hip dysplasia might be detected by using palpation when x-rays fail to identify malformations.) Early detection gives dogs better chances for normal lives without the need for total hip replacement.

Palpation is as much an art as it is a science. Sensitivity and keen observation contribute to the ability to successfully use palpation

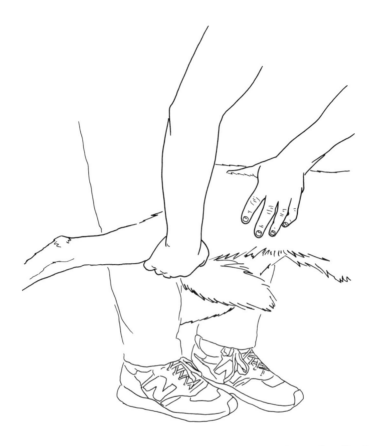

With the dog awake and in the standing position, palpation begins by allowing the dog to lean against your leg for support. Someone trained in the technique will palpate the hip by slowly extending the femur backward as fully as possible, paying special attention to the dog's comfort.

Illustration by Monique Raymond

techniques. A heavy touch will identify problems in hips that have progressed to a thickened joint capsule and chronic subluxation. However, to take full advantage of the palpation technique, a light touch is necessary to feel the subtle changes that the cup rim and joint capsule undergo in mild cases of dysplasia.

Backward Extension Test

The standard palpation technique for hip dysplasia diagnosis includes the backward extension test. Like the two-fingers test for elbow dysplasia, the backward extension test is quick and easy to perform by someone trained in the technique.

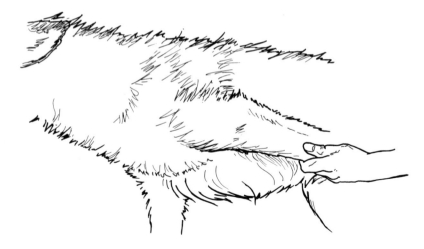

Pain or reluctance to display a full range of motion may indicate the area is a problem. Comparing the test on the opposite limb may help separate a painful area or verify the pet's natural resistance to palpation in general.

Illustration by Monique Raymond

With the dog awake and in the standing position, palpation begins by allowing the dog to lean against the person's leg for support. Palpating the hip begins by slowly extending the femur backward as fully as possible, paying special attention to the dog's comfort. The hip's range of motion is tested by using the femur as a lever. The leg should not be extended when holding the stifle because abnormalities in the stifle could lead to pain, which could be interpreted as originating in the hip joint.

Observe the dog's reaction to being handled. If the dog quickly rolls the pelvis away from the horizontal plane to avoid hip extension, become suspicious. Repeat the test with both hips and compare your findings from side to side.

PALPATING THE KNEES

The person begins by squatting or kneeling behind the dog and simultaneously cupping a knee in each hand. The palm of the tester's hand is held against the cranial aspect of the knee, and the fingers are held against the medial aspect. Feel for the general size, shape, and temperature of each limb; the findings should be the same from side to side.

Next, each knee should be palpated separately. With one hand cupping the knee as previously described, the other hand is used to bend and straighten (flex and extend) the leg. Care should be taken to

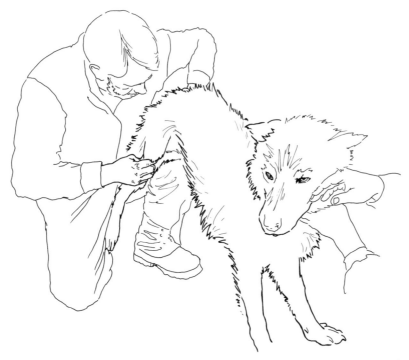

Palpating the knees is done by the examiner squatting or kneeling behind the dog, simultaneously cupping a knee in each hand. The general size, shape, and temperature of each limb should be felt.

Illustration by Monique Raymond

minimize the pain and be very gentle with the dog. The tester should not push or force the patella to move and should feel for any cracking, grating, or popping. Take special notice of the position of the patella (knee cap). It should smoothly glide in the groove formed by the femur.

If, either passively or with gentle pressure, the patella luxates (moves out of the groove) lateral or medial, a problem exists that needs to be evaluated. If the patella luxates, it may or may not cause pain (depending on the severity and chronicity), and it may or may not "pop" back on its own. If an intermittent luxation is suspected but not felt, a veterinarian should examine the dog a second time.

If the joint remains luxated following palpation, gently flex and extend the limb or allow the dog to walk it back in. Lateral luxations are usually very painful and traumatic in origin. Remember: Some luxations, if severe, remain constantly luxated and won't return to their proper site. Don't try to return a resistant patella to the site.

RADIOGRAPHY

If simple palpation suggests problems in the joints, a veterinarian will administer anesthesia and x-ray the joints to obtain an in-depth look at the areas. The dog may be sedated to obtain the correct radiographic position and to allow a manual examination of the joints. The x-rays may show irregular bone formations, calcium deposits, bone spurs, or other suspicious irregularities, which may confirm an orthopedic disease diagnosis.

For hip radiographs, the dog should always be sedated to allow proper radiographic position and palpation. The Orthopedic Foundation for Animals recommends that the dog be placed on its back with the pelvis symmetrical, with both femurs extended and parallel, and with the stifles rotated internally, placing the patellas on the midline. The radiograph should include the last two lumbar vertebrae and the stifle joints. It is essential, particularly in marginal cases, that the proper position and radiographic technique be obtained.

The radiographs may show abnormalities in the dog's structure, which will confirm any suspicions formulated during gait analysis or initial palpation. OFA radiologists are concerned with deviations in structure from the breed norm. Congruity and confluence of the hip joint are considered, along with subluxation, cranial acetabular margin, dorsal acetabular margin, craniolateral acetabular margin, acetabular notch, caudal acetabular margin, femoral head and neck, the presence of exostosis or osteophytes, and subchondral bone eburnation.

Certain factors can influence the findings seen on an x-ray, such as the age of the dog. The OFA will not evaluate or permanently grade hip x-rays of a dog under two years old. The OFA will examine and assign a temporary number to the x-rays of young dogs (less than two years of age). The reason is that x-rays of young dogs may misrepresent the true condition of the joint.

In addition to bone placement, joint laxity must be considered as vital information when assessing the hip joint. Often young dogs' radiographs can reflect good hips, when the hips are actually lax (at risk for dysplasia). A viable orthopedic exam of the hips must include evaluation of the laxity of the joint by employing PennHIP® or a similar technology such as stress radiographs.

Anesthesia may influence diagnosis because when dogs are fully relaxed they display true readings. Dogs not anesthetized may hold their hips tighter, giving inaccurate readings. Bitches in season often display greater laxity than they would normally; therefore, breeders should not wait until a bitch is ready to breed to have the hips evaluated. Periods of prolonged inactivity can cause subluxation; therefore,

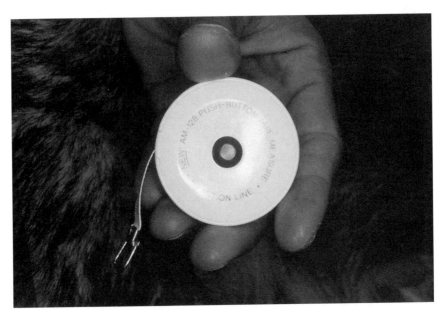

Use a tape measure to monitor muscle loss. Compare findings from side to side and keep notes. Repeat measurements periodically to assess trends.

dogs should be x-rayed when they are in good health and have good muscle tone.

Today, a variety of anesthetic agents are available for application in veterinary medicine. Although risks can be minimized by choosing appropriate anesthetics, a preoperative blood panel is recommended prior to administering anesthesia to ensure that the dog is a good candidate for withstanding anesthesia.

ANESTHETICS

Undergoing diagnostic procedures (such as radiography) may require administration of anesthesia. Fortunately for dogs and their owners, the risks of anesthesia have been minimized with the introduction of safe and effective agents. Dog owners should discuss the choice of anesthesia with their dogs' veterinarian and consider the costs associated with various agents in respect to the benefits delivered by each anesthetic choice.

Anesthetics are selected based upon health status of the pet, the breed (some breeds are more sensitive than others), the length of the procedure to be performed, and doctor preference. New drugs appear on the market quite regularly, and your veterinarian can provide you with current findings. However, many standard anesthetics are proven quite safe and effective. Among the commonly used agents are:

Injectable Anesthetic Agents

- *Acepromazine maleate* is most commonly used by general practitioners, but is contraindicated in dogs with epilepsy or seizures of any origin. The drug has proven excellent in calming animals, providing mild to moderate sedation that lasts from one to two hours.

- *Xylazine hydrochloride* is not commonly used because it impairs thermoregulation. The drug provides a moderate to deep sedation and analgesia for 20 minutes to one hour. Pets can display aggression upon arousal from this agent.

- *Diazepam (Valium)* is not suitable as a surgical anesthesia when used alone since it does not provide adequate anesthesia or analgesia.

- *Ketamine and Valium* are commonly used together for short-term immobilization. The drugs are limited to use in procedures lasting 5 to 30 minutes and have been known to produce seizures in rare cases.

- *Opioids* are not frequently used either alone or in combination. Opioids are excellent analgesics but poor sedatives.

- *Propofol* causes complete anesthesia and is most commonly used at referral or specialty practices. The drug is short-acting, smooth, complete, and provides quick wake-up times. Propofol is not currently licensed by the FDA for use in dogs.

Inhalant Anesthetics

- *Halothane* should not be used for restraint. The drug is long acting and requires a long wake-up time.

- *Isoflurane* is commonly used when complete anesthesia is required. It provides a quick, smooth wake-up within minutes of discontinuing the gas. Anesthesia continues for an unspecified length of time, as long as the gas supply to the animal continues.

NON-SURGICAL USES

Procedures other than surgery sometimes require the use of anesthesia. Isoflurane and Propofol are the preferred restraint drugs for palpation and radiographs when sedation or anesthesia is necessary. They allow an extremely quick, smooth, and safe wake-up. Although Propofol is an injectable and the duration cannot be controlled as precisely as Isoflurane, it is preferable to Isoflurane because an injectable is easier to administer and less stressful for the dog than an inhalant.

CONDITIONS THAT INFLUENCE LOCOMOTION

CHAPTER 6

GROWTH-RELATED LAMENESS

Who can resist the charms of an adorable puppy? Frankly, I've never seen an ugly puppy, and the very sight of a furry bundle of joy makes me lose my senses and forget my problems. This overwhelming puppy power inspires masses of people to think with their hearts instead of their heads, and puppies purchased on impulse make their way into millions of homes each year.

While many people receive satisfaction from these cute canines, others live to regret their impulses. Puppies purchased without consideration to genetic composition are at high risk of having congenital diseases, including developmental orthopedic diseases. Careful screening of breeding stock helps to control the incidence of disease, but problems can arise even in the best planned litters.

Some breeds are associated with specific limb and joint conditions, and owners of dogs in high-risk groups should be aware of the early signs of disease presentation. Early diagnosis and treatment is often the key to successful management.

Large and giant dogs are prone to lameness during the heavy growth period from 4 to 12 months of age. Included in this broad description are Rottweilers, German Shepherd Dogs, Great Danes, retriever breeds, Saint Bernards, Bernese Mountain Dogs, and Newfoundlands. Furthermore, some medium-sized dogs, such as Chow Chows and Australian Cattle Dogs, display growth-related lamenesses more often than others.

Small dogs are also not exempt from orthopedic problems. Congenital patella subluxation commonly occurs in various small terriers, spaniels, and Toy breeds. Chondrodysplastic breeds, such as Dachshunds and Basset Hounds, are prone to various stages of elbow dysplasia and premature growth plate closure.

GENETIC REGISTRIES

The Orthopedic Foundation for Animals (OFA) continues to be the watchdog for orthopedic soundness in breeding dogs, although others have introduced notable programs addressing orthopedics. The OFA's programs have expanded to cover a variety of diseases, such as the recent establishment of their elbow dysplasia registry.

Unfortunately, breeding dogs is not limited to the informed and ethical people. Furthermore, problems can occur even when every precaution has been taken. Breeders and scientists continue to research genetic issues, but until we have all the answers, dogs will be born predisposed to orthopedic illness. Repairing the errors of breeding is putting a Band-Aid on the problem, however, correcting an *individual* dog's orthopedic problem is possible with proper veterinary intervention. Most dogs with orthopedic problems can return to full function and maintain a high quality of life following treatment.

DIAGNOSIS

Veterinarians commonly encounter dogs with a disabling lameness. Many of these dogs suddenly exhibit extreme signs of joint disease, and their owners seek veterinary attention. Difficulty getting up or down, reluctance to walk on a lead, or noticeable limping may trigger an owner to seek a veterinarian's assessment of the dog's symptoms. An owner's astute observation of orthopedic abnormalities, promptness in obtaining an accurate diagnosis, and adherence to prescribed remedies offers the best chance for full recovery.

DIETARY CONSIDERATIONS

How much is too much? Follow your veterinarian's dietary recommendations for your dog. Don't *overfeed* or *over supplement*. Risk factors attributing to developmental orthopedic diseases, such as osteochondrosis, include a high dietary intake of calcium with a resulting imbalance of other minerals. High calcium intake has been associated with the development of wide retained cartilage cores, and irregularities in articular cartilage width. Diets high in protein may increase the growth lameness tendencies for large dogs because of growing too rapidly.

Your veterinarian may recommend a lower protein diet for puppies at risk. Large-breed dogs should be started on a diet consisting of approximately 21% to 24% protein at four months of age; small and medium breeds should be started at six months of age. At these ages, depending on the breed, the puppy *growth* diet should be discontinued. Dogs will grow to the same size as with a higher protein diet, just at a slower, safer rate. *Do not limit or give excesses of dietary protein, vitamins, or minerals without the advice of a veterinarian.*

ORTHOPEDIC DISEASES

Understanding the diseases that threaten our canine companions is important for disease prevention and treatment. Consider the diseases that threaten your breed.

Hip dysplasia, irregular formation of the coxofemoral joint, can affect dogs of any breed or size. However, large dogs are prone to the condition, and dysplasia affects some breeds with great frequency. Rottweilers, Golden Retrievers, Labrador Retrievers, German Shepherd Dogs, and Chow Chows are popular breeds with high incidences of hip dysplasia.

Canine hip dysplasia is an inherited disease caused by the interaction of multiple genes. According to the OFA, "No environmental *cause* has been found, but environmental factors may influence the degree of expression of the genes within an individual." Therefore, reducing the

Hip dysplasia, irregular formation of the cox-ofemoral joint, can affect dogs of any breed or size. In dysplastic dogs, the "socket" formed in the pelvis does not sufficiently hold the "ball" of the femur bone. Note degeneration in this area, which allows the ball to slip in and out of the socket and cause pain for the dog.

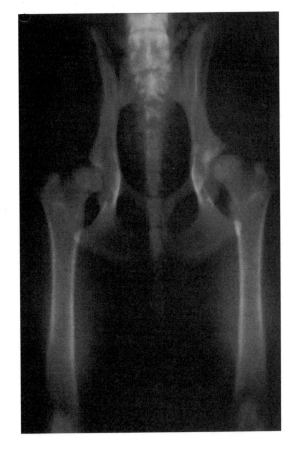

frequency of the disease is dependent upon selective breeding of dogs (and lines) with *normal* hips.

Early diagnosis provides options to treat the condition, therefore postponing/preventing further degeneration of the cartilage and severe joint damage. Radiographs (x-rays) of a dog's hips allow grading of acetabular depth, which may indicate dysplasia. However, experts recognize that hip dysplasia is affected by both acetabular depth and the degree of joint laxity, therefore palpation under anesthesia to assess the laxity is also important.

Radiographs have diagnostic limitations. Radiographs of young dogs' hips may not reflect subtle conditions that will become evident later in life. Some dogs with adequate cup depth depicted on radiographs eventually develop osteoarthrosis due to increased joint laxity (causing hip subluxation and labrum breakdown). Effective diagnosis of hip dysplasia requires consideration of palpation (assessing laxity) and radiographs (assessing cup depth).

Clinical signs of dysplasia become evident as dogs grow. Young dogs may not exhibit obvious signs of dysplasia, even though the condition may exist. Using palpation, veterinarians often can detect joint laxity when x-rays fail to identify bone malformations. *PennHip*®, a diagnostic procedure that is becoming widely used, relies on stress radiographs that provide a more accurate demonstration of hip joint laxity and thus improved diagnostic and prognostic abilities.

Surgery may often be indicated to correct dysplasia, and options vary from case to case. Triple pelvic osteotomy (TPO) or total hip replacement (THR) are commonly performed. Prognosis for a return to full function is excellent following either procedure. Femoral head ostectomy (removal of the femoral head) is a salvage technique for dogs under 24 pounds.

Medical management of hip dysplasia may not be a successful treatment option. It is a palliative option. In some dogs, depending on the severity of the dysplasia and the disposition of the dog, analgesics and the drugs adequan or cosequin may alleviate the dog's pain, but probably only temporarily.

The treatment of choice is surgical repair. The two most common surgeries are the **triple pelvic osteotomy** (TPO), which can be performed bilaterally (both sides) or unilaterally (one side only), and the **total hip replacement** (THR). The TPO is done by cutting the pelvic bone in three places and rotating the pelvis covering the femoral head to an angle that allows more appropriate coverage, thus preventing subluxation and degeneration of the joint. The THR is completed by removing the head of the femur and replacing it with a cobalt-chrome

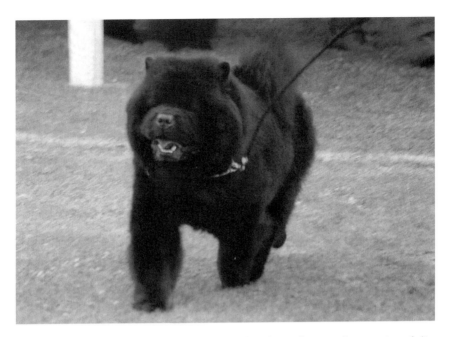

The degree of lameness in each leg may differ, depending on the severity of disease at each location and the pet's disposition or pain tolerance. A dog's tendency to pull or lean to one side while moving may indicate the location of pain.

prosthesis and then cementing an accompanying polyethylene plastic cup in the pelvic cup, giving the patient a new hip joint.

How does the surgeon choose the procedure for a given patient? Both surgeries are extremely successful when performed by a capable surgeon. The TPO requires that the surgical candidate's joint has not degenerated, thus it must be performed before arthritis occurs in the joint. The THR procedure is selected when the joint has degenerated and arthritis is present or if the joint is too loose and the pelvic cup would require rotation greater than 30 to 35 degrees. The patient must also be at least 11 months of age in order to ensure growth plates have closed.

Postoperative care for both surgeries requires two months of exercise restriction. Dogs are initially restricted to a crate and then slowly progress to gradual slow leash walks.

Osteochondrosis often causes transient and permanent lameness in dogs. Diagnosis of this condition presents challenges to veterinarians because this syndrome can be clinically silent, apparent only upon radiographic examination of the joint. Development of osteochondrosis occurs when a disturbance in the normal process of ossification results in cartilage cell nonresorption and replacement by bone. The persistent cartilage becomes necrotic and collapses. In the dog, most clinical cases are located in joints.

Historically, osteochondrosis was associated mainly with the shoulder joint. Today we include this disease among the causes of lameness involving the elbow, the hock, and, occasionally, the stifle.

Osteochondritis dissecans (OCD) refers to the stage of osteochondrosis when it becomes clinically apparent that the articular cartilage (which has thickened) has cracked, leading to the development of a cartilage flap. When left untreated, the chronic inflammation and loose cartilage bodies often lead to *degenerative joint disease (DJD)*, further crippling the affected dog. Prognosis for dogs with untreated OCD is difficult to make, due to the variable course the disease may take. Bilateral symptoms are often observed, or the disease may affect several joints.

The degree of lameness in each leg may differ, depending on the severity of disease at each location and the pet's disposition or pain tolerance. It is relatively common in large-breed dogs and is often bilateral. Therefore, if found in one limb, the symmetrical limb should always be evaluated as well.

Sometimes the onset of clinical signs is brought on by trauma or extreme exercise, which causes observers to miss the underlying *cause* or disease. OCD lesions do not always cause lameness, or the lameness may end spontaneously. For these reasons, although the flap will not reattach, some people feel pain relief and rest or pain relief and exercise will cause the flap to detach and hopefully move to a *cul-de-sac* in the joint. It is said this treatment can be attempted for three to six weeks.

The prevailing opinion is that surgery is the treatment of choice for OCD. In surgery, the flap and loose fragments are removed and the defect is smoothed by scraping. Surgical repair of OCD of the shoulder usually renders excellent results. Although it is still the treatment of choice, surgical results involving other sites are not as predicable. Postoperative radiographs can show that signs of DJD still almost always occur with OCD of the elbow, stifle, or tarsus. Although, the owners should remember that clinical lameness does not always follow.

OCD of the shoulder involves the caudal aspect of the humeral head and occurs more frequently in male animals. The shoulder is the most frequently diagnosed OCD site, and diagnosis requires observation of the dog's display of lameness and clinical evaluation (radiographs). Characteristic of this condition, lameness is worsened by rest, decreases with mild exercise, and worsens with heavy exercise. Pain is easily elicited by hyperextending the shoulder joint, and atrophy of the muscles may be apparent. A lateral radiograph of the extended shoulder joint will show a flattening of the contour of the humeral head in mild or early cases.

The shoulder is the most frequently diagnosed OCD site, and diagnosis requires observation of the dog's display of lameness and clinical evaluation by radiography. Lesions occur on the caudal aspect of the humeral head (joint surface).

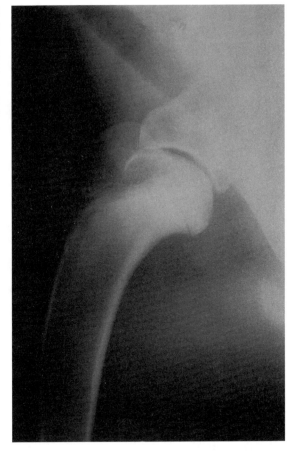

Early radiographic examination of the joint may not demonstrate a calcified cartilage flap. It may appear as a clear spot, and the fragment flap may not be visible. In such situations, contrast radiography (arthrography) may be necessary for definitive diagnosis. Arthrography is also recommended when people suspect joint mice (fragmented loose cartilage bodies) that are not easily visible. (Cartilage is not visible on radiographs unless mineralized or calcified.) Chronic cases of OCD may demonstrate radiographic evidence of osteoarthrosis. As the disease progresses, a mineralized cartilage flap may be observed on radiographs and the lesion will develop sclerotic margins.

Surgical treatment requires removal of loose cartilage and scraping of the lesion, followed by six weeks of on-leash exercise and physical therapy (passive flexing and extension of the joint and exercise including stepping on and off a short platform). Prognosis for the dog's return

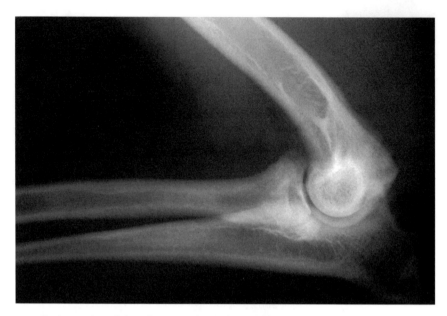

OFA radiographs of the elbow to check for dysplasia should be taken in extreme flexion. Note the periosteal reaction on the anconeal process.

to full function is usually excellent. During recovery, the defect is filled in by new growth.

OCD of the elbow occurs equally in both sexes. Pain can be elicited with extreme flexion, and dogs exhibit a limited range of motion. Joint enlargement occurs in chronic cases due to arthritic changes. Radiographs may appear normal early in the course of lameness, disguising the presence of the disease.

Follow-up views, taken three to six weeks after the initial radiographs, will show radiolucency on the weight bearing surface, with or without scaring of lesion margins. Surgery is the treatment of choice, and the coronoid process should also be carefully examined during surgical exploration of the joint. The prognosis is fair to good with early intervention.

OCD of the stifle is uncommon in the dog, however it can involve the lateral or medial femoral condyle, with the lateral being more common. Affected dogs exhibit pain during flexion or extension of the joint and often walk with the stifles flexed in exaggeration. This defect can be seen on an x-ray. Surgery is recommended for affected dogs. Removal of the cartilage flap and any free floating fragments will alleviate the condition.

OCD of the hock commonly involves the medial trochlea of the talus and is more common in male dogs. Rottweilers, Labrador Retrievers, and Australian Cattle Dogs are particularly at risk for OCD of this joint. Affected dogs hyperextend the hock and exhibit pain with forced flexion. Muscle atrophy of the limb may be present, depending on the duration of the lameness. Joint effusion is common, especially medially.

Oblique radiographs may be needed to show some lesions, especially those involving the lateral trochlear groove, which may occasionally be involved. Once again, surgical removal of the flap and any osteophytes is the treatment of choice.

Fragmented coronoid process (FCP) occurs when the medial coronoid process (of the ulna), a beak-like projection, becomes fragmented and causes joint pain. This commonly occurs with OCD in the joint. Lameness may be intermittent, may occur after rest, and may resolve after moderate use of the leg. Lameness intensifies following forced

OCD of the hock is more common in male dogs. Rottweilers, Labrador Retrievers, and Australian Cattle Dogs are particularly at risk for OCD of this joint. Note the irregular joint surface demonstrated in the radiograph.

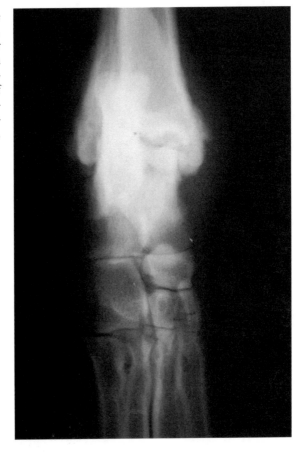

flexion of the joint, and physical examination may reveal restricted range of motion and crepitation.

FCP usually affects large breeds and may develop as early as six months of age. Some dogs don't show lameness until degeneration of the joint has occurred, which generally takes years. Once again, it is commonly bilateral. FCP can be a diagnostic challenge because the history and physical findings are often not specific and radiographs may not show the lesion. Therefore, palpation is usually the only consistent diagnostic tool.

FCP is difficult to see on radiographs. A slightly oblique view (25 degrees) is best. Most frequently, secondary changes will be seen. Exploratory arthrotomy may be necessary to confirm diagnosis.

Surgical treatment involves removing the loose coronoid fragment and is the treatment of choice. The prognosis is good if surgery is performed before significant degenerative joint disease develops.

Ununited anconeal process (UAP) results in the center of the anconeal process not joining with the proximal ulna. This developmental anomaly occurs most frequently in German Shepherd Dogs and is more common in males. The disease is also reported in large

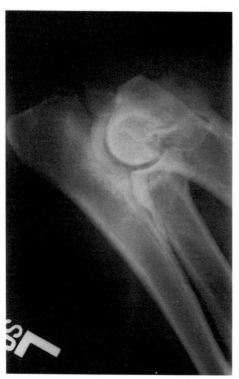

The anconeal process should unite before the dog is 5 months of age. Note its displacement in this 18-month-old German Shepherd Dog.

chondrodystrophic breeds, such as Basset Hounds and Bulldogs, but it is not a common condition. Lameness may be very subtle, increasing with exercise. Pain can be elicited with hyperflexion or extension of the affected limb. The dog often stands with the affected leg held in external rotation, with a shorter stride when moving.

Joint capsule thickening, joint effusion, and grating of joints are present in advanced cases. Complete fusion of the anconeal process (physeal closure) does not occur until 16 to 20 weeks of age. Therefore, diagnosis of a UAP should not be made before 5 months of age. A lateral radiograph in a fully flexed position will easily demonstrate the condition. *Bilateral UAP is approximately 30% in affected dogs.* Therefore, comparison films of both limbs should routinely be reviewed. When panosteitis is present, UAP may go unseen on x-rays, making inclusion of joint areas on the radiographs advisable.

Surgical treatment of displaced UAP involves removal of the anconeal process, which produces a good prognosis. UAP reconstruction may be considered, which results in improved joint stability. Occasionally, this disease is diagnosed later in life when chronic arthritis of the elbow joint is present.

Panosteitis is usually seen in dogs less than one year of age, but has been seen in older dogs. This is a spontaneous, self-limiting inflammatory disease of the long bones that commonly appears in young, fast-growing dogs. Males are more frequently affected than females. (Basset Hounds and German Shepherd Dogs are unique and occasionally develop this disease at one and one-half to two years of age.)

Lameness is acute and not usually related to trauma. Contributing causes include transient vascular abnormalities, allergies, metabolic disorders, stress, and autoimmune reactions *following* viral or bacterial infections. (Panosteitis has also been associated with von Willebrand's disease.) Females may have an incidence of hyperestrogenism with the first episode of the disease occurring in association with the first estrus.

Lameness may shift from leg to leg and may disappear without treatment. Deep palpation of the affected bone will elicit a painful response. X-rays may demonstrate an increased, patchy density of the cavity with a roughened surface. Radiographic signs may be present even after lameness has subsided.

Treatment is symptomatic with enteric coated aspirin and some limitation of activity. Clinical signs may continue for several months, usually resolving by one and one-half years of age. Prognosis is excellent, but it is wise to notify clients that lameness may shift to other limbs and may be intermittent for several months.

Legg-Calves Perthes disease (LCPD) (aseptic necrosis of the femoral head—osteonecrosis) occurs most often in small breeds and most fre-

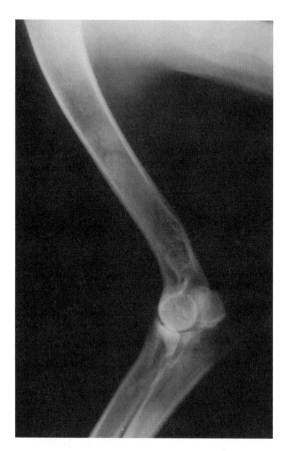

Panosteitis is a spontaneous, self-limiting inflammatory disease of the long bones that commonly appears in young, fast-growing dogs.

quently affects Wirehaired Fox Terriers, Miniature Pinschers, Miniature and Toy Poodles, Lakeland Terriers, West Highland White Terriers, and Cairn Terriers. When the disease is present, blood supply to the femoral head is cut off or lessened, and bone degeneration occurs. This may be of unknown origin or may follow trauma, for example, a fracture through the femoral neck.

The necrosis (bone degeneration) may eventually cause collapse of the femoral head, affecting congruity of the articular surface and predisposing the joint to secondary DJD. The process of LCPD can begin as early as three to four months of age; males and females are affected equally.

Affected dogs demonstrate subtle weight bearing lameness prior to collapse of the femoral head. Pain may be demonstrated by extension and abduction of the femur. Progression of the disease with development of DJD causes intermittent or continuous non-weight bearing lameness, muscle atrophy, and increased pain response on manipulation.

Early radiographic findings demonstrate increased lesions of the femoral head. Radiographs showing beginning changes may allow successful medical management of the disease; however, femoral head ostectomy is the accepted and usual surgical treatment. Most patients have already progressed beyond non-surgical treatment options by the time lameness occurs.

Non-surgical treatment consists of complete rest of the joint until radiographic lesions are no longer apparent. This entails strict crate confinement, with the dog being carried outside only for elimination and kept on a short leash during that time. This treatment course is usually four to six months. This is an amazingly long period of time for a puppy. Normal behavior and socialization may be compromised by confinement for that length of time.

A sling is *not* a treatment option. This causes severe and potentially irreversible damage to the muscles, bone, ligaments, tendons, and joint cartilage.

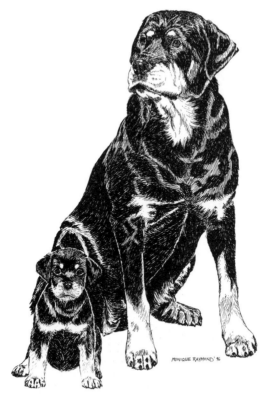

Selection of breeding animals based on genetic soundness promises a reduction in the number of dogs affected with orthopedic diseases.

Surgical repair consists of removing the head of the femur. This is the treatment of choice for LCPD. Because these dogs are generally so small, they regain excellent function of the hip (these dogs are generally too small for the THR prosthesis). In order to allow the hip to form a fibrous joint in the site of the ball and socket hip joint, physical therapy must be performed twice a day. This entails passive flexion and extension of the hip, starting within days of surgery and may be necessary for four to six weeks. It can be stopped once the dog is bearing weight on the limb.

If muscular atrophy has not occurred prior to surgery, a complete recovery usually takes 8 to 12 weeks. With cases involving atrophy, progress may evolve over the period of one year. Surgical success is excellent, and the patient does not require crate confinement.

SUMMARY

Dog breeders cannot become blind to orthopedic disease. Selection of breeding animals based on genetic soundness promises a reduction in the number of dogs affected with orthopedic diseases.

CHAPTER 7

DYSPLAS
(HIP AND

Hip dysplasia can affect dogs of any mix, breed, or size. However, la͏rge dogs are more prone to the condition, and dysplasia affects some breeds with great frequency. Rottweilers, Golden Retrievers, Labrador Retrievers, German Shepherd Dogs, and Chow Chows are popular breeds with high incidences of congenital orthopedic problems such as hip dysplasia.

What is hip dysplasia? It is the irregular formation of the coxofemoral joint. This is the joint that joins the femur, the longest bone in the body, to the hip socket. Dysplasia causes extreme pain for some dogs and significant discomfort for those mildly affected.

Hip dysplasia, a proven inheritable disease, involves multiple genes carrying the disease from generation to generation. Dogs can be carriers of some of the genes and not exhibit the disease, but when bred with another carrier, they can produce offspring that develop the disease. Breeders must monitor offspring and appropriately eliminate known or suspected carriers from their breeding stock to eliminate the disease.

The hip is a ball and socket joint, and the ball (femoral head) must fit well into the socket (cup) for the joint to function properly. The main contributors to the development of hip dysplasia are joint laxity and the depth of the acetabulum (cup). When joint laxity exists, the shallow cup allows the ball to pop in and out of place (subluxate) as the upward pressure exerted by activity pushes the ball over the dorsal rim of the cup. Abnormal wear and erosion occur both on the articular cartilage of the femoral head and the dorsal rim (labrum). The worn dorsal rim allows increased subluxation, and this degenerative cycle continues until severe secondary degenerative joint disease develops.

An owner may observe early signs of hip dysplasia, including:

- Reluctance to go up and down stairs or to jump

- Difficulty rising or lying down

- Bunny hopping when running (both hind limbs move together)

se or play intolerance

ference to lay or sit rather than to play

A change in attitude (associated with joint pain)

All of the above may be early signs of hip dysplasia.

DIAGNOSIS

Radiographs of a dog's hips are used to diagnose dysplasia. These pictures show the construction of the joint and allow the veterinarian to grade acetabular depth in dogs. Recently, however, experts have

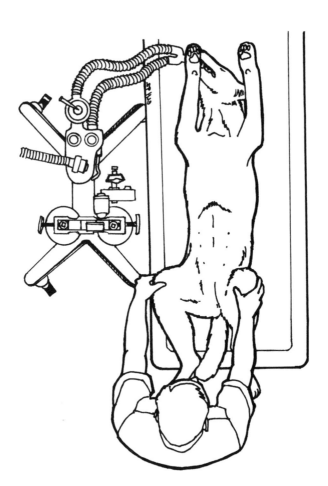

Effective diagnosis of hip dysplasia requires consideration of palpation assessing laxity and radiographs assessing cup depth.

recognized that hip dysplasia is affected by both acetabular depth and the degree of joint laxity.

Radiographs have limitations in diagnostics; radiographs of young dogs' hips may not reflect subtle conditions that will become evident later in life. Some dogs that show adequate cup depth on x-rays eventually develop osteoarthrosis due to increased joint laxity causing hip subluxation and labrum breakdown and leads to osteoarthrosis. Effective diagnosis of hip dysplasia requires professional palpation (assessing laxity) and radiographs (x-rays) assessing cup depth.

Clinical signs of dysplasia become evident as dogs grow. Young dogs may not exhibit obvious signs of dysplasia, even though the condition may exist. Using palpation, joint laxity can often be detected when x-rays fail to identify bone malformations. Early detection gives dogs better chances for normal life without the need for total hip replacement.

When deciding how to treat a dysplastic dog, you and your veterinarian must consider the age and size of the dog, the severity of the problem, and the dog's overall health. Diagnosis of dysplasia usually begins with a careful examination of the dog's movement at various speeds and under various conditions. A manual examination of the hip joint follows; a trained professional examiner can identify dogs with restricted movement, which *may* indicate dysplasia. Radiographs can confirm suspected dysplasia and identify the nature and severity of the affected joint or joints.

PALPATION

Palpation of a dog's hip and elbow joints takes only a few minutes, but can be extremely effective in detecting structural deformities. When palpating hips or elbows, the veterinarian assesses joint laxity, i.e., the tightness of the joint capsule, connective tissue, and fluid that comprise the joint. Palpation techniques are simple and can be performed as part of any veterinary examination.

Using palpation, hip dysplasia may be detected in young dogs, even when x-rays fail to identify malformations. Proper orthopedic examinations followed by radiographs (when indicated) can reveal structural problems in time to correct them before further joint degeneration occurs.

Throughout the procedure, keep the dog as comfortable as possible. Stand the dog and allow it to lean against you for support when necessary. Be sure to assess the dog's temperament prior to performing palpation; do not force palpation on a dog that is aggressive or in obvious pain.

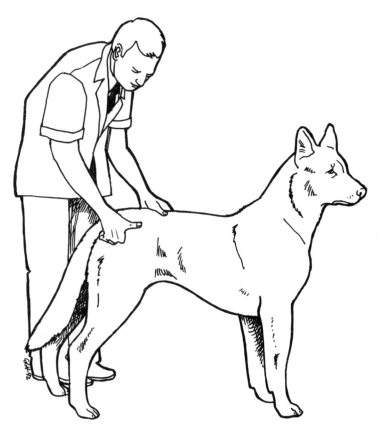

Palpation of a dog's hips takes but a few minutes, but it can be extremely valuable in detecting possible joint problems.

Backward Extension Test

With the dog awake and in the standing position, palpation begins by allowing the dog to lean against the tester's leg for support. Palpation of the hip is done by slowly extending the femur backward as fully as possible, paying special attention to the dog's comfort. Using the femur as a lever tests the hip's range of motion. The leg should not be extended when holding the stifle because abnormalities in the stifle could lead to misdiagnoses.

Observe the dog's reaction to being handled. If the dog quickly rolls the pelvis away from the horizontal plane to avoid hip extension, become suspicious. The test should be repeated with both hips; compare the findings between the two sides.

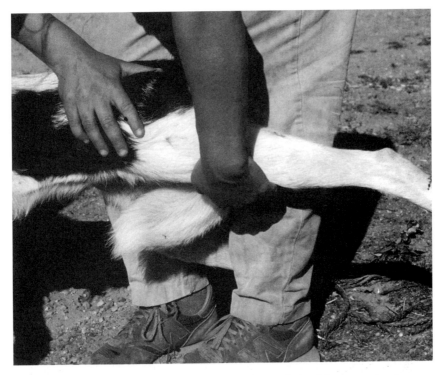

A backward extension test of a dog's hips can be performed by a veterinarian or a trained technician.

Palpation is as much an art as it is a science. Sensitivity and observation skills contribute to successfully using palpation techniques. A heavy touch will identify problems in hips that have progressed to a thickened joint capsule and chronic subluxation; however, to take full advantage of the palpation technique, a light touch is necessary to feel the subtle changes that the labrum (rim of the cup of the hip joint) and joint capsule undergo in mild cases of dysplasia.

Palpating Elbows

Elbow dysplasia is one of the most under-diagnosed conditions in dogs and has been found in significant numbers in 36 of 86 breeds that have evaluated by the Orthopedic Foundation for Animals. Because this condition is more common than previously thought, veterinarians must pay closer attention to the condition. However, initial screening need not be difficult or costly. Use palpation to assess your dog's elbow joint integrity.

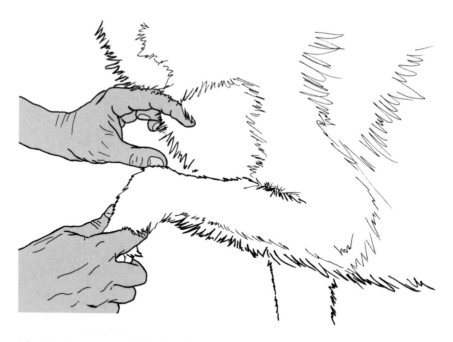

The distance measured in the elbow joint should be equal to the width of two fingers. Inability to bring the leg within the recommended width may signify instability.

Examination for elbow dysplasia begins with the two-fingers test. Carefully lift the front leg of the dog off the ground vertically. The foreleg is then gently but firmly pushed up close to the shoulder. The tester then holds the index and middle fingers together and places them between the point of the shoulder and the radial carpal joint as illustrated above. As the test is conducted, the dog is allowed to lean against the tester for support.

A dog with normal elbow structure will have a distance the width of two fingers between the point of the shoulder (greater tubercle) and the wrist joint (the point of radiocarpal articulation). The fingers should not slide down the angle, or else the reading will be inaccurate. A width greater than two fingers indicates decreased range of motion, which may indicate elbow dysplasia or osteoarthrosis of the elbow joint.

RADIOGRAPHY

If simple palpation suggests problems in the joints, a veterinarian should administer anesthesia and x-ray the joints to obtain an in-depth look at the areas of concern. Anesthesia enables the examiner to move the dog's hips into the correct radiographic position and allows a manual examination of the hip joints. The Orthopedic Foundation for Animals recommends that the dog be placed on its back with the pelvis symmetrical, with both femurs extended and parallel, and with the stifles rotated internally, placing the patellas on the midline. The radiograph should include the last two lumbar vertebrae and the stifle joint. It is essential, particularly in marginal cases, that the proper positioning and radiographic technique be obtained.

The radiographs may show abnormalities in the dog's structure, which will confirm any suspicions made during gait analysis or initial palpation. OFA radiologists are concerned with deviations in structure from the breed norm. Congruity and confluence of the hip joint are considered, along with subluxation, cranial acetabular margin, dorsal acetabular margin, craniolateral acetabular margin, acetabular notch, caudal acetabular margin, femoral head and neck, presence of exostosis or osteophytes, and subchondral bone eburnation. The most important of which are shallowness of the acetabulum, secondary degenerative changes of the acetabulum and femoral head, and coxofemoral subluxation. Joint laxity, a major factor in the development of hip dysplasia, may not be apparent using standard radiographs.

Certain factors can influence the reading of x-rays. Joint laxity may not be determined; a joint may appear normal on a radiograph, but actually be loose. Young dogs (under two years of age) may x-ray better than they will at maturity.

Anesthesia may influence diagnosis; when dogs are fully relaxed they display truer readings. Dogs not anesthetized may hold their hips tighter, giving inaccurate readings. Bitches in season often display greater laxity than they would normally; therefore, breeders should not wait until a bitch is ready to breed to have the hips evaluated. Periods of prolonged inactivity can cause subluxation; therefore, dogs should be x-rayed when they are in good health and have good muscle tone.

When purchasing a puppy, ask to see the OFA certificates for *both parents*, especially if purchasing a large-breed dog. *Although OFA certification cannot guarantee that the puppies will be clear of dysplasia,* it demonstrates that the breeder has taken steps to reduce the chances of dysplasia in the litter.

TREATMENT OPTIONS

What if your dog is diagnosed with dysplasia? When should surgery be performed? According to Gail Smith, VMD, Ph.D. of the University of Pennsylvania School of Veterinary Medicine, there is no clear-cut rule as to when surgery is the recommended course of action. Dr. Smith says, "Veterinarians often disagree on this subject, and the concerned dog owner should seek second opinions if they are considering hip surgeries." Consultations with veterinarians who specialize in orthopedics (board-certified orthopedists, Diplomates, or Fellows of the American College of Veterinary Surgeons) are recommended.

If your dog has been diagnosed with hip dysplasia, you must consider the options for treating the condition and make decisions regarding the dog's future. Dysplasia is a serious, crippling disease, but it is treatable. Most dysplastic dogs can live full, active lives following appropriate surgery.

Veterinary orthopedic surgeons routinely perform two procedures for correcting hip dysplasia: triple pelvic osteotomy (TPO) and total hip replacement. The preferred surgery for a given patient depends on many variables. However, young dogs are the best candidates for TPOs. TPOs cost about half as much as total hip replacements, and the procedure is less taxing. TPOs must be performed before arthritis develops in the joint.

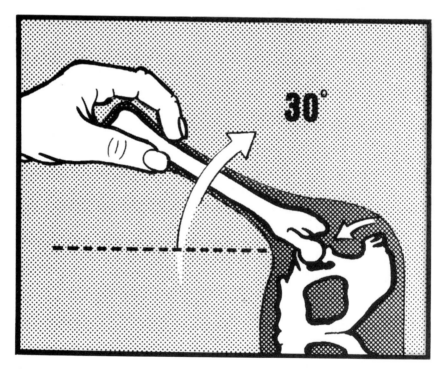

If a dog's joints reduce at angles of 30 degrees or less, owners should strongly consider TPO as a corrective surgery.

When diagnosis of hip dysplasia occurs before osteoarthrosis has developed, the dog may be a candidate for triple pelvic osteotomy. If the dog's joints reduce at angles of 30 degrees or less, strongly consider TPO. This angle is measured by examining the flexibility and position of the joint while the dog is anesthetized.

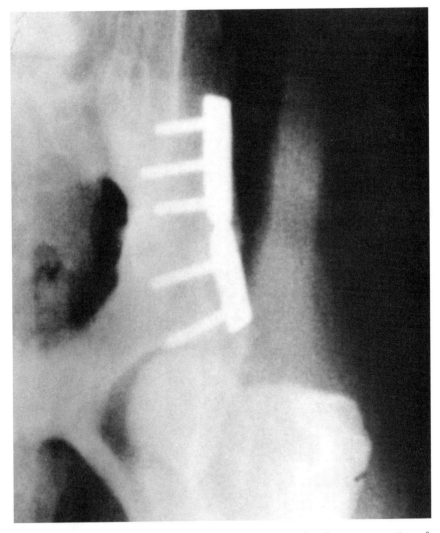

Hip of a dog that has had triple pelvic osteotomy. Note that the reconstruction of the pelvis has altered the hip joint so that more than 50% of the ball of the femoral head now fits into the cup of the acetabulum.

TRIPLE PELVIC OSTEOTOMY

This is an effective procedure that changes the orientation of the dog's hip socket, providing extended coverage of the femoral head by the socket. Young dogs with shallow acetabulums are ideal candidates for TPO. This procedure can be performed on one or both hips. When both hips are recommended for correction, they can be done simultaneously. Hospital stays for TPO patients are short, typically three to seven days.

TOTAL HIP REPLACEMENT

This procedure has been in clinical use for more than 15 years. Total hip replacement is recommended for dogs older than 11 months of age

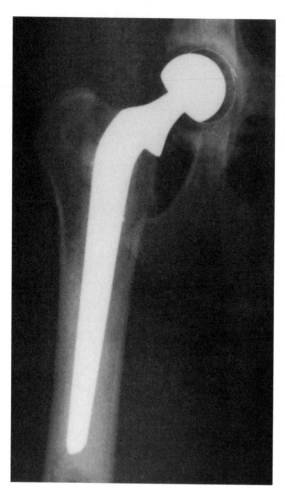

Hip of a dog that has had total hip replacement. A cobalt-chrome ball and rod have replaced the dysfunctional femoral head of the dog, and a Teflon cup has replaced the deformed cup of the hip, allowing for return to full function.

Hip of a dog that has had femoral head and neck resection. The head and neck of the femur were removed. This procedure is considered inferior to triple pelvic osteotomy or total hip replacement, but can provide relief from the pain associated with hip dysplasia. Dogs may suffer limited return to function with this procedure.

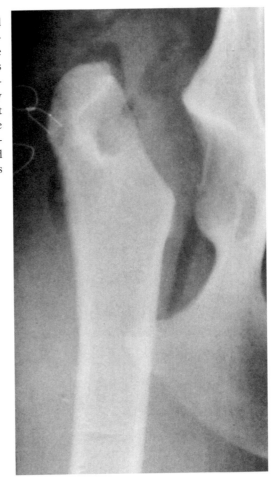

whose hips reduce at angles of 30 degrees or more, or that exhibit evidence of osteoarthrosis. This procedure is very effective and offers return to normal activity to most dogs. Those who have undergone the procedure are pain and limp free with dramatically improved mobility.

Approximately 80% of dogs will need only one hip replaced. Many dogs, even working dogs, return to full activity after total hip replacement. Pet owners have reported great satisfaction with total hip replacement in their dogs. Representative cases have been followed for more than 10 years with no difficulties reported in the sample.

FEMORAL HEAD AND NECK EXCISION

With this procedure, the femoral head is removed, allowing a false joint to form. The procedure may sustain small dogs, but is less desirable for large dogs. The cost of this surgery is significantly less than other procedures, but the prognosis for return to full function is guarded. Dogs who have undergone femoral head and neck excision may be able to walk through the house, but are unlikely to want to jog several miles or jump repeatedly to catch a ball.

MEDICAL MANAGEMENT

The treatment of choice for hip dysplasia is surgery, but if need be, medical management can be attempted to alleviate pain. Medical management consists of analgesics and anti-inflammatory drugs, exercise restriction, and weight control. Reasonable expectations of these would be to alleviate pain, maintain joint function, slow degenerative changes, and allow daily function. Eventually, medical management will not allow a satisfactory life, due to the progressive nature of canine hip dysplasia.

The decision to perform surgery should never be made lightly, but your veterinarian can help you choose what's right for you and your dog. Careful selection of a surgeon is necessary to ensure the best results. Use the same criteria you would in selecting a surgeon for yourself. Is he or she a board certified specialist? Ask the veterinarian about his or her experience with the recommended procedure. Ask for references or to see dogs who have undergone the procedure under discussion. Does the surgeon offer guarantees for the work?

RECOVERY

Freedom from pain and the opportunity to lead full, productive lives is possible for most dysplastic dogs. Recovery time varies, but pet owners are often surprised by their dog's ability to recuperate quickly from major surgery. Following any surgery, however, you may need to confine your dog or exercise it on a prescribed schedule. Your cooperation is necessary for the dog's optimal chance for a full recovery.

Of course, the best treatment for this or any disease is prevention. Screening breeding stock is the key to preventing the spread of this inherited disease. However, for dogs that are stricken with dysplasia, surgery is available to allow these dogs to return to full, active lives.

SELECTIVE BREEDING

Twenty years ago, very few dog owners could pronounce dysplasia, let alone pose questions to their veterinarians about cause, prevention, and treatments of the disease. Thanks to educational efforts within the veterinary community, today's informed pet owner understands the disease process and accepts responsibility for ensuring that their dogs avoid needless pain and suffering.

Breeders have been actively striving to eliminate the condition through selective breeding. Progress has been seen in many breeds, but others are still struggling to overcome alarming percentages, particularly in large and giant breeds. What causes the condition? Experts may disagree, but most concur that popularity and an increased market for puppies encourage unknowledgeable people toward indiscriminate breeding of animals not thoroughly screened. However, even in pedigrees displaying multiple generations of breeding stock that have undergone radiographic screening and been found free from dysplasia, puppies continue to develop hip dysplasia at alarming rates.

THE ORTHOPEDIC FOUNDATION FOR ANIMALS (OFA)

Responsible breeders screen dogs for congenital defects before they are bred. This screening includes x-raying the dogs' hips for evaluation, especially in breeds with a high incidence of the disease. The x-rays are graded by a team of veterinarians, and each dog is rated as excellent, good, fair, borderline, mildly dysplastic, moderately dysplastic, or severely dysplastic. *Dogs diagnosed with dysplasia should not be bred.* Furthermore, their close relatives should be suspected as potential carriers of the disease and be eliminated from breeding programs when possible, or judicially bred and carefully monitored.

The OFA has identified the following breeds as having the highest incidences of hip dysplasia: Bulldog, Boykin Spaniel, St. Bernard, Bullmastiff, Newfoundland, American Staffordshire Terrier, Bloodhound, Field Spaniel, Fila Brasiliero, Chesapeake Bay Retriever, Bernese Mountain Dog, Kuvasz, Mastiff, Golden Retriever, Giant Schnauzer, Rottweiler, German Shepherd Dog, and Chow Chow.

Although the breeds mentioned above have exhibited high incidences of dysplasia, other breeds may actually be more heavily affected. When reading these statistics, one must consider that the OFA can only base this data on x-rays submitted to them for evaluation. This group of dogs is not a representative sample of dogs in general; it only includes dogs owned by responsible breeders thought to have a chance of passing the screening. *Obviously, x-rays of dogs clearly exhibiting dysplasia are not submitted for evaluation.* Furthermore, dogs in puppy mills, most pet dogs, and mixed-breed dogs' x-rays are not submitted for evaluation and are therefore not represented in the statistics.

The OFA aims to reduce, if not eliminate, cases of hip dysplasia in all dogs. Toward this end, The American Kennel Club, the Morris

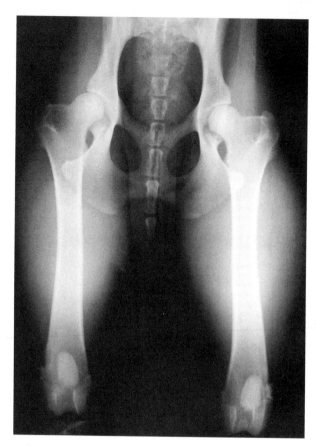

More than 50% of the femoral head (ball) fitting into the joint cup indicates normal hips.

Animal Foundation, and the OFA are supporting a research project at Michigan State University and the University of Michigan under the direction of Dr. George Brewer. The study involves DNA technology and aims to determine the genotypic status of individual dogs who are potential breeding stock.

The OFA recommends that owners look for their dog's breed on the incidence list to see what the chances are of hip dysplasia developing. It is this book's authors' opinion that if the breed is high on the list, don't procrastinate. Ask your veterinarian to palpate and x-ray your puppy at six to eight months of age, while you can still prevent or reduce the crippling arthritis that accompanies hip dysplasia. Don't delay if your dog is older than eight months of age.

"Early diagnosis and treatment may prevent the pain and arthritis that accompany dysplasia. Early diagnosis also increases the number of available treatment options. Some of the surgical procedures must be done prior to the development of arthritic changes," according to the OFA.

Less than 50% of the femoral ball fitting into the joint cup indicates dysplasia.

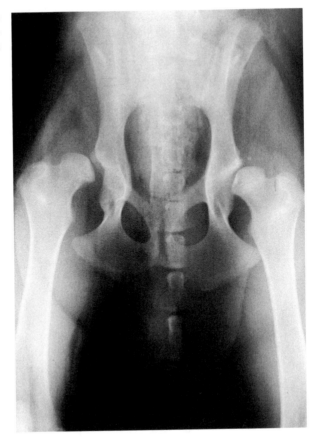

PennHIP® (University of Pennsylvania Hip Improvement Program)

—Elizabeth LaFond, DVM
Post-doctoral research fellow in the laboratory of Dr. Gail Smith

The primary reason hip dysplasia is a concern to dog owners, breeders and veterinarians is that the arthritis often occurring as a part of the disease can cause significant discomfort and/or impair a dog's function. Arthritis does not occur in very young dogs; it develops after a dog has walked on loose and unstable hips for a long period of time. Evidence of hip arthritis on radiographs of a dog (in the absence of a history of trauma) is confirmation that the dog has hip dysplasia. The question is, can we tell which dogs are more likely to develop hip arthritis *before* it shows up on x-rays?

In 1983, Dr. Gail Smith, a veterinary surgeon and bioengineer from the University of Pennsylvania School of Veterinary Medicine, began to take another look at canine hip dysplasia and to address the question of early assessment of canine hips. He began by investigating the long-held belief that joint looseness (laxity) plays a major role in the development of arthritis. The idea behind this theory is that if a dog's hips have excessive laxity, then, as the dog walks, runs and jumps on the joints over time, there may be excessive wear. The body attempts to compensate for the excessive wear and laxity by trying to stabilize the loose joints. Unfortunately, the result is the development of often painful and sometimes debilitating arthritis.

The PennHIP veterinarian is trained and certified to take radiographs of a dog's hips in such a way as to reveal the maximum amount of joint laxity. For the x-ray, the femoral heads (the "ball" part of the ball-and-socket hip joint) are pushed out of the acetabula (the "socket" part) as far as they will easily go while the dog is under sedation with all its muscles relaxed. A Distraction Index (DI), which does not depend on dog breed, size and shape, can then be calculated from the x-ray. The DI is an objective measure that corresponds to the percent of potential movement of the femoral head within the acetabulum.

Dr. Smith and his colleagues conducted many tests to determine the best way of performing this technique and to assess the relationship between the laxity readings veterinarians could get with this method and the subsequent development of hip arthritis. The research behind the PennHIP method spanned ten years and included both biomechanical and clinical testing. Very briefly, the major findings are:

BIOMECHANICAL FINDINGS

- *Hip position is very important for detecting laxity.* How much laxity will be seen on the x-ray is heavily dependent on the position of the dog's legs when the radiograph is taken. The maximum amount of laxity is seen when the hips are in the same position a dog uses while standing normally (neutral position). The traditional position used for evaluating hip status has the dog lying on its back with its legs stretched straight out (as if it were a person lying down). Testing shows that the amount of laxity seen in this position is much less than that seen in the neutral position.

- *Measured laxity is consistent among examiners.* The biomechanical behavior of the canine hip is such that even if two veterinarians push the femoral heads out of the acetabula with different amounts of force, they will actually get very similar readings in the amount of laxity they can detect.

CLINICAL FINDINGS

- *DI is consistent over time.* Dogs have essentially the same amount of laxity at 4 months of age as they do at 2 or 3 years of age.

- *Tighter hips are better hips.* Breeds of dogs known to be free of hip dysplasia (such as performance Greyhounds and Borzois) have uniformly tight hips. Even within known dysplastic breeds, those dogs with very tight hips are not susceptible to developing arthritis; the looser the hips are, the higher the risk for arthritis.

- *Arthritis susceptibility is breed-dependent.* Different breeds of dogs have different tolerances to laxity in their hip joints. For example, given the same amount of laxity, a German Shepherd Dog is more likely to develop arthritis than a Rottweiler. The theories for these differences are under investigation.

- *Non-genetic factors play an important role in arthritis expression.* Not all dogs with loose hips will necessarily go on to develop arthritis. Environmental factors can dramatically influence the expression of arthritis in susceptible dogs. Because of this environmental influence on the expression of arthritis, laxity alone, in the absence of clinical signs, is not yet a recommended indication for surgical intervention. However, knowledge of hip laxity may be very helpful in guiding the management of and expectations for the dog.

- *Hip laxity is inherited.* Tighter hipped parents tend to produce tighter hipped puppies. (For more on the heritability of hip laxity, see Chapter 13.)

- *The PennHIP method is safe.* The PennHIP procedure to measure hip laxity has proved to be safe and effective even when performed multiple times on the same dog.

In summary, the PennHIP procedure is a reliable, sensitive, and safe method of measuring hip laxity in dogs. Furthermore, the laxity it measures is a very good indicator of the risk for developing hip arthritis. All veterinarians that perform the PennHIP technique are trained in the scientific principles behind the method and have completed certification exercises to assure uniformity.

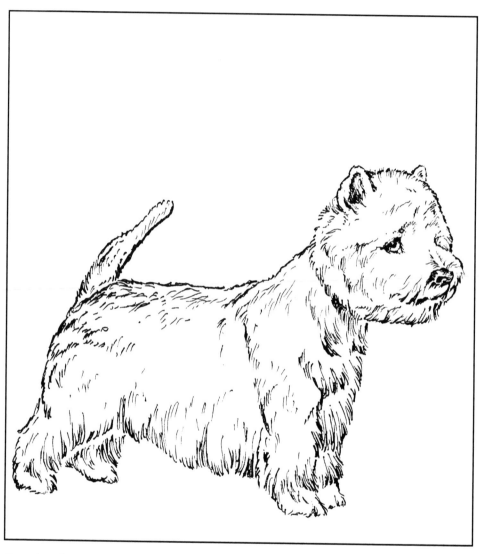

Dogs less than 30 and more than 60 pounds may be more at risk for knee problems. Small dogs sometimes suffer from slipping stifles (luxating patellas), while larger dogs can experience ruptures of the cruciate ligaments.

CHAPTER 8

CONDITIONS
AFFECTING THE KNEES

The knee (patella or stifle) of the dog is a movable joint that interconnects the femur (thigh bone) to the tibia and fibula (shin bones). The knee joint also contains three smaller bones; the patella (or kneecap) and two small sesamoid bones.

The patella, or kneecap, is the largest sesamoid bone in the body. It is somewhat round and curved to join with the femur, forming a functioning joint. The patella is embedded in the tendon of the quadriceps muscle, which extends the length of the femur. The tendon attaches the patella to the tibia. This complicated joint is stabilized by a number of tendons and ligaments. Of the ligaments, the most commonly discussed in veterinary medicine are the cruciate ligaments—the anterior (cranial) cruciate ligament and the posterior (caudal) cruciate ligament.

The cruciate ligaments form an x–shaped apparatus that runs from the front of the joint to the back. The ligament that runs from the back of the joint to the front is called the *anterior cruciate* ligament, while the ligament from front to back is the *caudal cruciate* ligament. The anterior cruciate ligament controls internal joint rotation and prevents hyperextension of the joint, as well as limits cranial displacement of the tibia. The posterior cruciate ligament limits caudal displacement of the tibia and aids in the control of internal rotation and the prevention of hyperextension. Neither cruciate ligament can limit external rotation of the tibia.

Rupture of either cruciate ligament can occur, but rupture of the anterior cruciate ligament is much more common. Rupture of this ligament allows for abnormal rotation of the joint, as well as allowing abnormal movement of the long bones forward and backwards upon each other. The result of this instability on the health of the joint can be severe. This will be discussed in a later section.

This x–shaped structure is critical to the stability of the joint, as it prevents the two major long bones (the femur and the tibia) from moving too far forward or backward. This also allows the joint to twist on its long axis without dislocating. The ligaments are subject to rupture when the stress is overbearing, such as that sustained in a sudden turning movement or from a blow to the joint.

The stifle also contains fibrocartilagenous disks, each called a meniscus. These crescent-shaped discs, wedged between the surfaces of the femur and the tibia, function as shock absorbers (protecting the articular surfaces). They also increase the stability of the knee, aid in joint lubrication, and act as "washers," allowing incongruities between the joint surfaces to exist without causing damage.

The functions of the ligaments, menisci, muscles, and joint capsule play a vital role in the ability of the stifle joint to hinge or glide on its axis.

The knee joint can be compared to a hinge on a door. The door and the building frame represent the two major long bones (femur and tibia), while the hinge represents the knee joint. The pin that holds the hinge together is like the cruciate ligaments. If the weight of the door is proper for the size and construction of the hinge, the door can function normally within its frame for many years. If, however, the door is too heavy for the size and construction of the hinge, then the door may sag or fall away from the frame and not function properly. Forcing the door to operate under these conditions results in damage to the door, the frame, and/or the hinge. Obviously if the pin is removed from the hinge, the hinge may fall apart, unless you are very careful, because it is unstable.

This is quite similar to what can happen in the knee joints of large, heavily muscled, and fast-growing dogs.

RECOGNIZING KNEE ABNORMALITIES

An active dog can injure this joint quite easily. Working in the field exposes the dog to irregular surfaces, creating the possibility of tripping in a hole or getting tangled in brush. Slick surfaces, startling noises, or roughhousing with other dogs can also expose dogs to the potential for injuries. However, obesity, conformation deformities, and repeated stress to the joint are most commonly responsible for stifle injuries, especially cruciate ruptures.

Large dogs are susceptible to ligament ruptures, while small dogs are affected by patella abnormalities. How can you recognize knee injuries? When dogs avoid using the back legs, throw their weight to the front legs, occasionally skip in movement or display pain, there may be abnormalities in the knee joint, and an orthopedic examination is indicated.

Other preexisting orthopedic problems contribute to the rupture of cruciate ligaments. When dogs feel pain in one joint, they shift weight to other joints. Often the knee bears responsibility for weight bearing in dogs with other degenerative joint diseases. Owners who postpone addressing conditions such as hip or elbow dysplasia often find themselves treating cruciate ligament ruptures in addition to the dysplasia. Again, *early treatment of joint diseases decreases severity and minimizes pain for the dog.*

EXAMINATION

Dog owners can perform *some* components of the stifle exam at home. If the outcome of an examination leads the examiner to believe that the dog may have a stifle problem, the exam can be augmented by a veterinary evaluation.

A general lameness exam should be completed as the initial step when examining a dog for a stifle problem. During this observation phase, you should look for a few specific things. Dogs with stifle problems may stand with a bowlegged or knock-kneed posture. A dog with bilateral problems may shift weight to the front legs, changing the normal 60/40 weight distribution. Quite often when a dog suffers a ruptured anterior cruciate ligament (RACL), the medial meniscus is damaged. The damaged meniscus may make an audible click when the dog walks. This can be very loud and obvious, and it does not take a trained ear to hear.

The next two steps, palpation and manipulation, can reveal further diagnostic data. Patience is definitely a virtue while palpating the stifle joint in that frequently the changes are subtle and time must be taken to get a good feel of the joint. (We're not sure who needs more patience, the dog or the examiner!)

Manipulation of the stifle should be conducted at the veterinary hospital. It frequently necessitates the use of sedation or anesthesia to relieve pain or anxiety and thus tensing of the muscles (or biting), preventing disclosure of the existing joint dysfunction.

Palpation can best be accomplished with the dog in a standing position. The examiner squats or kneels behind the dog, simultaneously palpating both stifles. The palm of the hand cups the cranial aspect of the stifle, the fingers wrap medially. Using this method, gentle palpation can be accomplished, and very minor or subtle differences can be appreciated. Chronic stifle instability leads to fibrous thickening of the joint capsule on the medial side. This can easily be missed if careful, slow, comparative palpation is not performed. Prominence of the cranial aspect of the tibia usually goes unnoticed if both stifles are not palpated simultaneously. Both these findings suggest anterior cruciate ligament rupture. You should assess swelling, heat, or pain in the joints at this time. Once again this information is best established by simultaneous palpation.

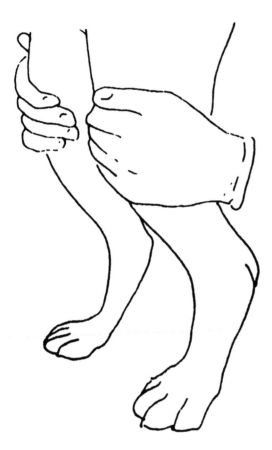

Dogs with stifle problems may stand bowlegged or knock-kneed. A dog with bilateral problems may shift more weight to the front legs, changing the normal 60/40 weight distribution. Quite often when a dog suffers a ruptured anterior cruciate ligament, the medial meniscus is damaged. The damaged meniscus may make an audible click when the dog walks. This can be very loud and obvious and does not take a trained ear to hear.

Next, the location of the patella is determined at rest and during motion by gently flexing and extending the knee. (Initially, the relationship of the patella in the joint must be established during weight bearing.) Also take the time to palpate the rest of the limb, looking for abnormalities such as muscle atrophy, pain, or swelling.

Manipulation of the stifle joint should be done with the dog laying on its side with the knee to be examined uppermost.

Most manipulations are most successfully performed by a veterinarian and frequently under sedation or anesthesia, but the overall nature of the joint can be assessed by a careful and gentle technician. The joint should be manipulated through a complete flexion and extension, noting the range of motion. Also note pain, instability, or crepitus (crepitus is best described as a cracking, crunching, or popping that is sometimes heard but usually felt).

Dependent upon the results of the observed gait analysis, palpation, and manipulation, the owner and veterinarian may follow up with radiographs, contrast arthrography, synovial fluid examination, arthroscopy, or other exploratory surgery.

X-rays of the stifle joint (as with the hip or any joint) are limited because they cannot show joint instability (stress views secondarily identify joint instability). They also cannot diagnose a ruptured cruciate (the cruciate cannot be seen on radiographs), but they can provide important information and are an essential addition to manipulation and palpation. Radiographs evaluate the extent of degenerative changes, demonstrate avulsions or neoplastic conditions, help differentiate between fluid-induced or soft tissue swelling, and offer an abundance of information about bone conformation and abnormalities, especially associated with growth-related disease or genetic patellar luxation.

Plain radiographs do not allow evaluation of soft tissue structures. Injection of a contrast agent with x-rays (contrast arthrography) outlines the joint capsule and structures within the joint. Soft tissue abnormalities may sometimes be defined in this manner.

Evaluation of the synovial fluid differentiates between inflammatory and non-inflammatory joint conditions, such as arthritis and immune mediated disease.

Arthroscopy is examination of a joint through a scope using very small incisions, unlike those used in regular surgery. Although commonplace in human medicine for both diagnoses and treatment, the procedure has not yet replaced exploratory surgery in the dog.

MEDIAL AND LATERAL PATELLA LUXATION

Patella (knee cap) luxation, a frequent occurrence in dogs, manifests in different types of luxation and varying grades of severity. Understanding the causes and effects of this problem allows dog owners to make educated decisions about the care of pets.

When the patella is normally positioned, the cartilage surface of the patella glides smoothly and freely along the trochlear groove. However, dogs affected by patella luxation experience a "popping out" of the patella as the knee attempts to function. The affected dog may cry out in pain, or it may just manipulate itself and adjust the kneecap back into position.

Medial patella luxation can be present at birth (congenital and possibly indicating a genetic condition) or acquired. The condition affects both dogs and cats and can be unilateral (occurring on one knee) or bilateral (affecting both knees). Patella luxation is classified and graded according to severity, and the severity can increase in time, due to repetitive stretching of soft tissue causing skeletal deformities.

Dogs in early stages of the disease experience minimal discomfort, but as the disease progresses, the patella "popping" causes intense pain for the dog. Therefore, many dogs do not suffer lameness until adulthood, when they may have been harboring the disease for many years. In middle- to older-aged pets, 15 to 20% of the cases presented exhibit concurrent rupture of the cranial cruciate ligament. Help is available for dogs affected by patella luxation. Good diagnostic and surgical practices have produced a 90 to 95% success rate for achieving active and pain free use of the patients' affected limbs.

Medial patella luxation is one of the most common stifle problems seen. The genetic (inherited) form of the disease commonly occurs between four and six months of age in Toy and Miniature breeds of dogs and other small breeds, including Miniature and Toy Poodles, Yorkshire Terriers, Lhasa Apsos, Chihuahuas, and Pekingese. Although clinical signs sometimes present earlier, they usually are not evident until later in life. Congenital medial patella luxation is characterized by a bowlegged stance and a pulling on the patella when the dog is in motion.

Trauma-induced lateral patella luxation is a relatively rare condition that may occur from minor skeletal or mild patella instability. Luxation induced by trauma is usually lateral but may occur medially. Lateral luxations occur more frequently in large dogs, and unlike the medial dislocations (luxations), clinical signs are accompanied by acute inflammation and severe pain. The affected limb will not bear weight, and swelling often occurs. Anesthesia may be necessary for palpation of the patella, and radiographic examination can rule out other injuries to the stifle joint.

LATERAL PATELLA LUXATION

Lateral luxation in large dogs is often seen in the breeds that are affected by hip dysplasia, including Rottweilers, Golden Retrievers, Labrador Retrievers, Chow Chows, and German Shepherd Dogs. Research has shown that congenital hip dysplasia deformities may cause this condition.

Lateral patella luxation can cause deformity of the femoral head, due to the rapid growth seen in large breeds. Genetic (and possibly nutritional) factors are keys to the development of this condition. Clinical signs occur around five to six months of age with a thickening of the stifle joint tissues and a knock-kneed and/or a cow-hocked stance with the toes pointed out. In cases with associated hip dysplasia, the correction of both abnormalities is necessary to prevent progressive deformities.

CLASSIFICATIONS OF MEDIAL PATELLA LUXATION

Preliminary classification of patella luxation is important in order to evaluate the patient. These grades (1 being the least severe, 4 being the most severe) are based on the pet's stance, movement (gait), and how easily the veterinarian can manipulate the patella.

Grade 1

Occasional carrying of the leg is seen, often described as skipping or hopping, which may be transient, often returning to normal by itself. Your veterinarian may easily luxate the patella manually and return it to its normal position. Pain may be evident only when the kneecap is luxated.

Grade 2

The frequency of luxation increases, becoming more or less permanent. The pet will usually carry the leg, but will occasionally bear weight on it. When palpated by the veterinarian, a dry, crackling sensation (crepitation) may occur in the joint. A grade 2 luxation can increase in severity and, if not surgically treated, can develop into degenerative joint changes.

Grade 3

Permanent dislocation is seen, although weight bearing may still be possible (however, the stance will appear somewhat crouching or bow-legged). Surgical intervention should not be delayed, especially if this is found in a young, growing dog. Rapid growth of abnormalities results in progressive deformities.

Grade 4

Permanent luxation is seen, with the affected limb always carried, creating a bowlegged, crouching stance. Early surgery is strongly recommended at this stage for bony deformities of the femur and tibia.

DETECTING LUXATION

Early detection of patella luxation is critical for providing a good quality of life. In addition to the pain and suffering caused by the knee abnormalities, approximately 95% of dogs with patella luxation have a related structural abnormality. If these conditions are treated when the dog is young, progressive deformities can be avoided.

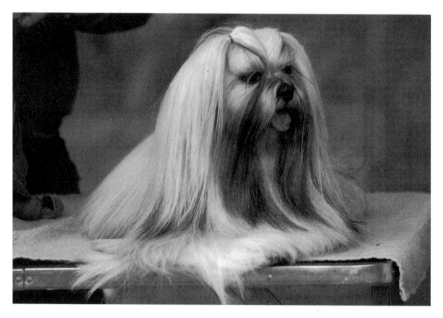

Owners of small dogs, like this Lhasa Apso, should have their dogs' knees examined while the dogs lie on their sides. This can be performed in conjunction with regular veterinary examinations.

Routine veterinary examinations should include evaluation of the joints with particular attention paid to those dog breeds known to be predisposed to orthopedic abnormalities.

TREATMENT

In early to mild stages, soft tissue reconstruction may be sufficient to correct the problem. Increasing degrees of luxation, duration, and multiple joint involvement require a variety of bone reconstruction techniques, with soft tissue repair often being necessary.

Luxating patellas can be surgically corrected to allow a dog to lead a productive life free from pain. The key to successful treatment lies in early diagnosis and therapy.

RUPTURE OF THE CRUCIATE LIGAMENT

The anterior cruciate ligament is a very important structure in the knee (stifle) joint of the dog. This ligament helps strengthen and stabilize the knee joint, allowing its normal range of motion. Rupture of the anterior cruciate ligament is one of the most commonly encountered orthopedic injuries in dogs and results in joint instability that leads to inflammation and damage to the articular cartilage of the joint.

When damaged, the cartilage begins to degenerate, leading to changes in the underlying bone, which is the beginning of arthritis and can lead to permanent disability of the joint. The inflammatory changes begin almost immediately, and the degenerative changes can be apparent within one week after injury. It is, therefore, critical that ruptured anterior cruciate ligaments be repaired and the joint stabilized as soon as possible.

Rupture of either cruciate ligament can occur, but rupture of the anterior cruciate ligament occurs most commonly. Rupture of this ligament allows for abnormal rotation of the joint as well as abnormal movement of the long bones forward and backward upon each other. The results of this instability on the health of the joint can be severe and can cause dogs so much pain as to prohibit weight bearing on the affected leg.

Dogs with acute rupture cannot place weight on the joint and show swelling, pain, and joint instability. Dogs with chronic injuries may occasionally refuse to put weight on the joint, but will demonstrate muscle atrophy and will have palpable bone spurs. A meniscal "click" may be heard by the owner.

Large-breed dogs, especially those with heavy musculature, present a high incidence of this cruciate rupture. Among the most commonly affected breeds are Newfoundlands, Akitas, Bulldogs, American Staffordshire Terriers, Rottweilers, Boxers, and Labrador Retrievers. Weight appears to be a significant risk factor, and dogs with a body weight of greater than 50 pounds are primary candidates for anterior cruciate ligament ruptures. Owners and breeders of large dogs should be aware of the condition and its causes, diagnosis, and treatment.

RECOGNIZING RUPTURE

Rupture of the anterior cruciate ligament can be due to acute injury or chronic degeneration, which can completely sever or can partially tear the ligament. Regardless of severity, dogs with ruptured ligaments require surgical correction of the condition, because it is always progressive and will always become more severe.

Acute rupture is usually due to traumatic injury, such as an automobile accident. These dogs display severe lameness and may carry the leg to avoid putting weight on the affected joint. The joint often appears swollen and may be very painful if manipulated. Dogs may protect the leg and will try to avoid physical examination. Dogs may

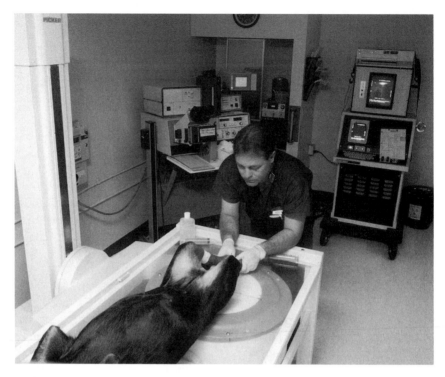

Radiographs may not show evidence of existing knee damage, however, bone scans (being performed on this two-year-old Rottweiler) and MRIs (magnetic resonance imaging) can provide greater access to the soft tissue structures in the joint.

become aggressive as a result of pain, so caution should be used when examining injured dogs.

More commonly, rupture of the ligament is thought to be due to chronic degenerative changes in the ligament, perhaps again due to the strain of carrying a heavy load in large, heavily muscled dogs. In more chronic cases, the lameness may be less severe than in the acute ruptures and may appear to improve slowly with time. In rare cases, lameness resolves completely, however, discomfort may recur with age and the development of arthritis in the affected joint. Degenerative tears are sometimes difficult to diagnose because lameness tends to be less noticeable. A partial degenerative tear can also lead to the development of arthritis over time.

Your veterinarian can diagnose rupture of the anterior cruciate ligament by physical examination of the joint and with x-rays. The veterinarian will consider the "drawer sign" as diagnostic for a ruptured anterior cruciate. The drawer sign is abnormal forward movement of the tibia relative to the femur which is held in a stable position.

How can you determine that a cruciate rupture is causing pain and lameness rather than another condition? X-rays eliminate fractures or other injuries as causes of lameness in acute ruptures, and they can identify degenerative or arthritic changes associated with chronic ruptures. New technology, such as bone scanning and magnetic resonance imaging (MRI), can be useful for confirming rupture or partial tearing of the anterior cruciate ligament in great detail and with more success.

TREATMENT OF ANTERIOR CRUCIATE LIGAMENT RUPTURE

In the large, heavily muscled breeds, the knee joint should always be surgically stabilized after rupture of the anterior cruciate ligament. Many surgical techniques exist for repair of the ligament and/or stabilization of the joint. The technique chosen by a veterinarian may depend on his or her training and experience and may vary according to the size of the dog or the duration of the injury.

Regardless of the technique, the goal of surgery is to stabilize the joint and prevent the abnormal movement that results in degenerative

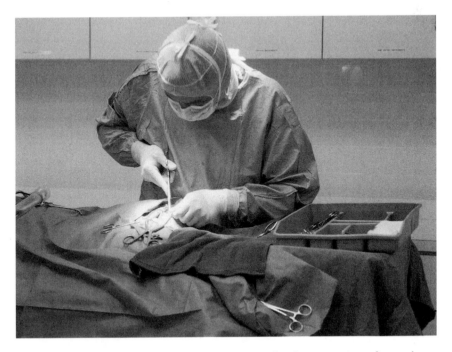

Surgical procedures provide excellent prognoses for the correction of most knee abnormalities.

change and, ultimately, arthritis. Most techniques involve either repair of the ligament, replacement of the ligament (with grafted tissue or an artificial material), or augmenting a partially torn ligament. Surgical repair will usually reduce lameness and lessen degenerative changes in the joint, thus delaying or preventing the onset of arthritis. However, in large dogs, a surgically repaired knee may never be as strong as it was before injury. A torn meniscus is also removed at surgery.

Medical treatments with anti-inflammatory drugs (such as enteric coated aspirin) may help relieve pain and inflammation. Drugs for combating degenerative changes in the cartilage and preventing arthritis are under development.

CONCLUSION

Hind leg lameness of sudden or slow appearance should alert the owner to the possibility of anterior cruciate ligament rupture. A veterinary examination can confirm the presence of this common injury. Prompt diagnosis and repair can prevent the development of arthritis, improve the dog's quality of life, and perhaps extend the life expectancy of the dog.

CHAPTER 9

COMMON JOINT DISEASES

Joints, the hinges of the body, allow bones to move at angles to each other, thereby producing movement potential. Function and movement of the dog depend on proper function of the joints.

Joints (arthroses) in the dog vary in composition and function. The ball and socket joint, represented by the shoulder and hip, is probably the best known joint formation in the dog. The dog's knee (stifle) moves in two directions, but has no rotational capability. Hinged joints, such as the elbow and knee joints, move on one axis. The carpus (wrist) and tarsus (ankle) represent a simple gliding or plane joint, with limitation in movement based on a sliding motion.

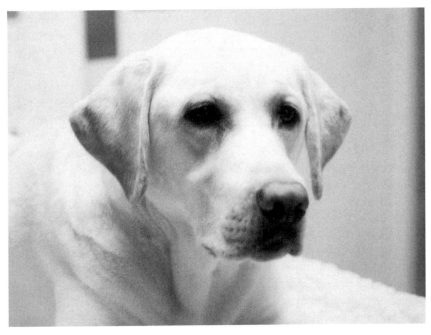

Function and movement of the dog depend on proper function of the joints.
Photo by Leslie Bird

119

Understanding basic mechanical aspects of the joints allows inter-pretation of movement and assessment of orthopedic soundness. Most joints of concern in canine orthopedics are synovial joints. The synovial joint structures include the *joint cavity, capsule, synovial fluid,* and *articular cartilage.* Other structures involved in joint movement include ligaments, and fibrocartilage pads. A change in joint structure alters the range of motion. Restoring the original range of motion can be ham-pered by muscles, ligaments, the joint capsule, and the shapes of the bones involved.

Healthy dogs enjoy fluid movement, brought about by properly functioning joints. Diseased or injured dogs may possess the desire to perform "normal" activities, but are often limited by their dysfunctional joints. However, joint damage is repairable, although an ordeal we would rather avoid.

RECOGNIZING PROBLEMS

Joint disease is usually categorized as degenerative (non-inflammatory) or inflammatory. Although all types of joint disease or trauma cause inflammation, this terminology is used because the inflammation in degenerative or traumatic joint disease is not the primary cause of the deterioration, which it is in inflammatory joint disease.

Inflammation causes pain in the joints, and arthritis is the term commonly applied to such conditions. *Arthritis can be degenerative or inflammatory.* Inflammatory arthritis can be further divided into *infectious* or *immune* (non-infectious or sterile) inflammation.

Joints can be influenced by environment, but genetics often con-tributes to joint instability. Early detection and correction of joint abnormalities offer the best prognosis for the joint to return to full function.

However, complete reversal of pain or dysfunction is rarely achiev-able in dogs with joint disease. Control is usually more likely than cure. In cases where surgical repair is possible, the clinical benefits increase dramatically with early diagnosis and treatment. The earlier the treat-ment, the less secondary damage to the joint (caused by inflammation, instability, and/or infection) can occur. Degeneration of a joint cannot be reversed, but can be halted, and some remodeling can occur, which will help the joint function properly and, hopefully, free from pain.

Dogs with inflammatory joint disease associated with systemic signs, such as rheumatoid arthritis or systemic lupus, have a poorer prognosis, but with appropriate therapy they usually can live a func-tional, albeit quiet, life.

It is important that the owner and veterinarian work together in selecting treatment modalities for a dog. In order to minimize frustration and obtain the best possible outcome, the pet owner must understand the expectations or limitations of therapeutic choices when dealing with joint disease. It cannot be stressed enough that *the earlier appropriate care is given, the better the prognosis.*

DEGENERATIVE JOINT DISEASE (DJD)

Probably the most common joint disease seen in veterinary medicine, this slowly progressive form of cartilage degeneration is usually caused by trauma or abnormal wear on the joint. It is frequently considered the result of an abnormal stress placed on normal cartilage or normal stress acting on abnormal cartilage. DJD is classified as primary (ideopathic or no known cause) or secondary (a known predisposing cause or injury exists).

The cause of primary DJD has not been identified. Secondary DJD is associated with abnormal joint mechanics or direct trauma to the articular cartilage. The collapse of the joint space leads to a remodeling of the bone underneath the cartilage (the subchondral bone). These changes lead to inflammation of the synovial membrane with fibrous tissue forming around the joint. This leads to the development of osteophytes, small outgrowths of bone on the joint margins. This process of degeneration begins within seven days of joint injury.

Osteoarthrosis (DJD) is manifested by clinical signs of pain, stiffness, and decreased range of motion. Obesity can contribute to the development of DJD by placing additional stress on joints. Rest and confinement may relieve some of the pain, and controlled exercise in the form of slow walks or swimming is important to maintain joint mobility and muscle mass. Weight control is important for pets with severe osteoarthrosis.

When a pet's activity has been reduced, it is important for owners to reduce dietary intake as well. Sympathetic feeding can contribute to joint disease. DJD is rarely seen in young dogs and is best treated through preventive measures and changes in the pet's environment.

Analgesics may be used to alleviate pain. Drug therapy is adjusted to the individual's needs, but (when possible) alternate-day or as-needed therapy is preferable to a daily dose.

In the case of secondary DJD, not only are rest, confinement, and drug therapy helpful, but finding and treating the underlying cause should be the goal, preferably before the DJD becomes moderate or severe. Early surgical treatment of the underlying cause is the treatment of choice for secondary DJD, although the possibility of a less-than-ideal outcome of surgery should be anticipated. The return to full function is not always possible, and long-term analgesics and weight control may be needed in conjunction with surgery.

Common underlying causes of secondary DJD are trauma, ruptured cruciate ligaments, developmental diseases (such as hip or elbow dysplasia), ununited anconeal process, fragmented coronoid process, osteochondritis dissecans, and patella luxation. Obviously, the most successful outcomes occur when the underlying cause is surgically repaired before DJD has occurred.

INFLAMMATORY JOINT DISEASE

As with degenerative joint disease, inflammatory joint disease can be classified into two groups: disorders caused by an infection and those that are non infectious, usually immune-mediated inflammation. The noninfectious group can be divided into erosive disorders (rheumatoid arthritis) and nonerosive (systemic lupus erythematosus). All of these conditions cause pain, but the erosive disorders also deform the joints.

Unlike most orthopedic problems, which cause a discrete lameness, inflammatory joint disease usually involves multiple joints and thus tends to cause a stiff or stilted gait. Furthermore, systemic signs of illness often accompany inflammatory joint disease. Affected dogs may exhibit fever, anorexia, and a reluctance to walk.

Blood work and joint fluid analysis, along with x-rays, are usually necessary to differentiate between infectious and immune-mediated joint disease. But even these findings can be difficult to interpret because the predominant findings in both disorders stem from the inflammation and thus can be similar.

Treatment for infectious joint disease involves selecting medication for the specific agent involved. Treatment for autoimmune or noninfectious joint disease relies on immunosuppressive drugs. *Because immunosuppressive drugs would allow an infectious disease to flourish, it is very important to differentiate between the two disorders before treatment.* If the testing does not differentiate between the two, it is best to treat for an infectious origin for three to five days. If no response, then treat for immune-mediated disease.

Surgical intervention is not reasonable for most patients because inflammatory disorders usually involve multiple joints and the pathological progression cannot be halted by surgery.

IMMUNE-MEDIATED ARTHROSES

Animals affected by immune-mediated joint disease are usually mature, and the disease frequently involves more than one joint. Further disease classification may be considered based on the presence or absence of resultant joint deformity caused by erosion of synovial structures.

Rheumatoid arthritis (RA) is a slowly progressive inflammatory joint disorder. Although considered rare in dogs, when present it is generally found in middle-aged and older animals. Pronounced joint instability and deformity usually affecting the carpus, tarsus, and feet often accompanies the disease. The digits are often deformed, with the feet turning out. Joint swelling is caused by an inflammation of the soft tissue, with decreased quantities of synovial fluid found in affected joints.

Prognosis for complete cure is poor, but some comfort can be achieved with medical therapy of corticosteroids or other immunosuppressive agents. Weight control is important in the treatment of RA.

Plasmacytic-lymphocytic synovitis is an erosive inflammatory joint disorder that affects small- and medium-sized dogs. The stifle is the most commonly affected joint, and bilateral joint laxity and instability usually characterize the disease. Difficult to diagnose, this condition is commonly mistaken for a ruptured cruciate, with the true diagnosis made only during surgical exploration.

Surgical findings include thickening and discoloration of the synovial joint membrane or an abnormality in joint fluid. Treatment with immunosuppressive drugs should be withheld two to three weeks post-operatively to allow for primary healing of surgical sites. (Immunosuppresive and cytotoxic drug therapy can increase the risk of infection and poor healing of the surgical site.)

Systemic lupus erythematosus (SLE) most commonly affects the joints, muscles, skin, and kidneys. In SLE, the immune system inappropriately produces antibodies against the DNA material inside the cells. Manifestations of this disease are dependent upon the location of the cells affected, and diagnosis of SLE is often difficult.

A blood test is available to detect the antibodies directed against the DNA (anti-nuclear antibodies: ANA test), but this test often produces false readings. Environmental, infectious, hormonal, and drug reactions have all been identified as possible causes. Corticosteroid and cytotoxic drug therapy is the treatment of choice, and treatment specific for other body systems affected must occur concurrently.

Clinical remission of this uncommon disease can be achievable, but often for only short periods of time.

Idiopathic nondeforming arthritis affects large breed adult dogs, and is the most common form of immune-mediated, nondeforming arthritis.

Multiple joint involvement is common with an acute onset of lameness. The gait is often stiff or stilted. The cause of this type of arthritis is unknown, thus the term idiopathic. It may be related to an immune hypersensitivity associated with various conditions including infections, gastrointestinal disease, and neoplasia. Idiopathic, nondeforming

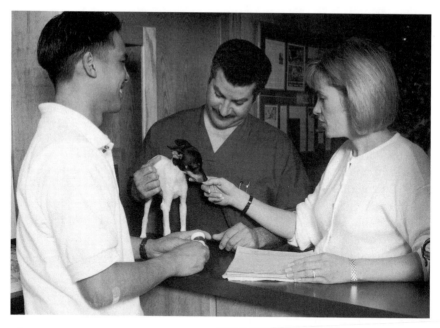

Plasmacytic-lymphocytic synovitis, an erosive inflammatory joint disorder, affects small- and medium-sized dogs, such as this Toy Fox Terrier.   *Photo by Leslie Bird*

arthritis is generally treated with corticosteroids or in combination with cytotoxic drugs. The response to treatment is often dramatic, with remission dependent on the type of associated condition.

INFECTIOUS JOINT DISEASES

A variety of infectious forms of joint disease, including bacterial, rickettsial, fungal, and viral, threaten dogs. Differentiation between these forms is based on patient history, physical signs, examination of fluid from affected joints, systemic blood testing, and x-rays.

Bacterial arthritis occurs infrequently, mostly in young, large-breed dogs. Involvement of a single joint (the hip, shoulder, stifle, or elbow) is more common than multiple joint involvement. This infection is usually associated with a penetrating injury or underlying immune suppression. Puppies can become infected from uterine or mammary gland infections, with multiple joint involvement and a generalized septic arthritis. Rapid onset of lameness and infected, swollen joints that are warm and painful to the touch are seen.

Joint fluid analysis (with a culture of the bacteria) and sensitivity testing (to show which antibiotic the bacteria responds to) is recommended if infection is suspected. Treatments include antibiotics, lancing and draining of affected joint(s), and in septic conditions where the infection is in the bloodstream, monitoring of the lungs, liver, and kidneys for distant organ involvement should be performed.

Surgical draining of the joint may become necessary and can greatly alleviate pain. Successful treatment depends on early intervention.

Bacterial endocarditis, an infection affecting one or more valves of the heart, can spread from the heart to other body organs and to the joints. Multiple joints can become infected, producing a generally stiff gait. Lameness may also result from muscle inflammation, and successful treatment of bacterial endocarditis is difficult. Long-term intravenous and oral antibiotics are needed to manage this disease.

Rickettsial and *spirochete associated arthritis* are caused by organisms carried by specific ticks. Rocky Mountain spotted fever, ehrlichiosis,

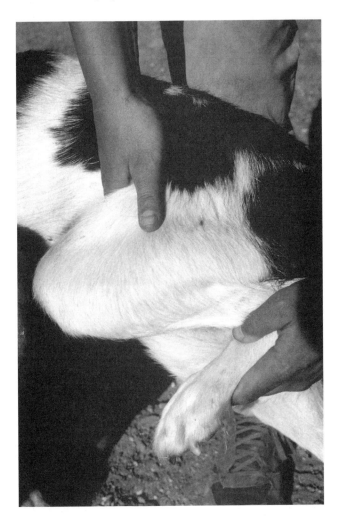

Joint swelling and pain can signify fungal arthritis.

and Lyme disease are caused by these organisms, and each can be associated with joint pain. These diseases also are able to cause other nonspecific and diverse signs, which can make diagnosis difficult.

The specific organisms are not usually identified on joint fluid analysis, and diagnosis is based on clinical signs, history of animal habitat, the ruling out of other disease causes, and response to therapy. Antibodies to the organisms can be detected with a blood test, but only after two to three weeks of infection. (The blood tests must be repeated two to four weeks apart to demonstrate a rising titer.) The diseases are treated with tetracyclines.

Fungal arthritis infrequently occurs in dogs, however when present, it is usually the result of an extended fungal infection from bones. Microscopic evaluation or culture of joint fluid can often show the organisms. Treatment involves the use of one or more antifungal medications and must be continued for months or years.

CONCLUSION

Whether surgical or medical options are employed in the treatment of canine joint disease, many important factors are common to the treatment of all joint diseases. These include rest, physical therapy or exercise therapy, and weight control, which can be as important to the success of treatment as the primary option itself.

CHAPTER 10

SPINAL (VERTEBRAL) COLUMN DISEASES

Anyone who has ever witnessed the speed and grace of an athletic dog can appreciate the complexity of moves and the ability to react quickly. Herding dogs must stop, turn, and drop with split-second timing. Police dogs must be able to instantly change postures from mild-and-relaxed to ready-to-attack. Even family pets react to their environmental needs. Consider the Sheltie that chases birds in the backyard and the Keeshond that alerts owners to someone approaching the front door. All actions require a dog to be in overall good condition, but they especially require a healthy, pain free, flexible back, a "normal" back.

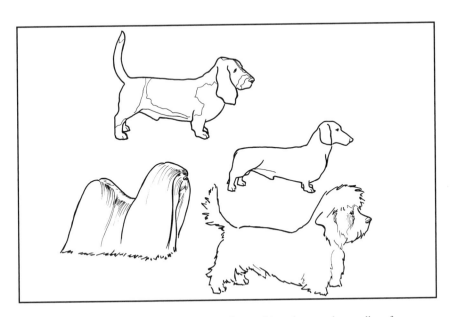

The intervertebral disks, elastic formations that cushion the vertebrae, allow for movement and protect against shock and related traumas. Breeds commonly affected by diseases of the spinal column include those with long backs and short legs. Clockwise; Basset Hound, Dachshund, Dandie Dinmont Terrier, Lhasa Apso.

Illustration by Monique Raymond

The vertebral column is not only the supporting structure of the body, but it also carries the nerves that move muscles, allow sensation, tell you where your limbs are without having to look, and guide the whole system. The spinal cord is part of the complex computer that runs the body. All dogs depend on a healthy spinal cord to perform routine acts.

How does a dog react quickly enough to perform athletic feats? How can the animal think quickly enough to send messages from the eyes to the brain, to the feet or head? Just as a ballerina or figure skater knows "instinctively" where she is during a spinning move, or how we know just how far to lift our feet when going up a flight of stairs, dogs know the correct placement of their feet, head, and tail by relying on the outer part of the spinal cord, which controls peripheral knowledge. Motor and reflex actions, sensation, and pain are also governed by this incredible mechanism, the spinal cord.

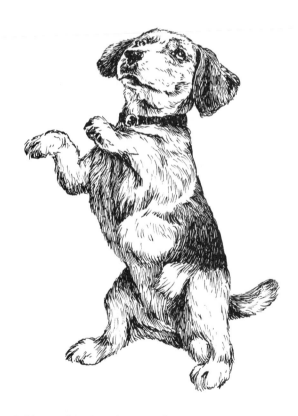

Stressful activities, such as jumping onto furniture, flex the spine at extreme angles and heighten the possibilities of dogs rupturing disks.   *Illustration by Chris Hoy*

Your dog could not walk or stand without the spinal column. All physical activities depend on the proper function of the spine and the nervous system it protects. Without a working nervous system, the brain cannot send messages to other parts of the body. For example, the dog's feet wouldn't know to move and it would not respond to touch or pain.

However, aging and disease can slow dogs down. The older dog that previously raced up the steps takes them one-at-a-time. A puppy's gait seems not quite right—a little wobbly, not like other littermates. Suddenly a six-year-old Cocker whimpers and stares at the owner, communicating discomfort caused by simply standing up.

Care of the spine, like all good medical plans, requires preventive measures to keep the back healthy and corrective options when problems occur. Of course, an ounce of prevention is worth that pound of cure, so in respect to backs, physical fitness is pure gold. (Keeping a dog at the proper weight is important.)

Selective breeding of dogs is critical to eliminate back diseases. Breeders of dogs that are predisposed to developing back diseases must carefully consider the genetic history of dogs in their breeding programs. *A dog with genetic back problems should not be bred*—even if it's the cutest, nicest dog you've ever known. Furthermore, breeders must consider the blood relatives of the dogs they breed and the medical history of the dogs in that line. A breeder should be able to discuss the dogs in several generations of a pedigree, knowing each dog's strengths and weaknesses as well as what relatives have produced and paying close attention to medical aspects of the dogs.

What does a "normal" back look like? The answer varies quite a bit, and knowing your dog's breed Standard will give you the answer. A few dogs, such as the Greyhound, should have a roached back, a back that curves upward when the dog stands still. The German Shepherd Dog's back should demonstrate an obviously sloping topline (the line drawn from the shoulder to the tail). However, most dogs should have a straight back, or a topline that slopes slightly downward toward the tail.

Your dog, regardless of breed, should give the impression of strength and comfort during all activities. A dog that appears uncomfortable, lazy, or in pain should receive a thorough veterinary examination.

Keeping the back healthy is an important goal of all vertebrates (animals with backbones, including humans). Human medicine has called attention to this important element of health care, and workers' compensation cases document that the back is easily injured when proper care is not given. Dogs depend on healthy backs to support their bodies, to allow them to function normally, and to maintain a healthy immune system.

BACK BASICS

The back is made up of two basic components: the *vertebral column* and the *spinal cord*. The vertebral column is a bony support system with a canal in the center. The spinal cord is a thick trunk of nerve tissue that extends down the spinal canal from the base of the brain to the pelvic region.

Dogs, being vertebrates, have a physical structure that is tied together by this vertebral column, or spine. The spine serves a very important function in the dog; it protects the spinal cord and roots of the spinal nerves, aids in the support of the head and the internal organs, and furnishes attachment for the muscles, ribs, and pelvis.

The vertebral column is made up of bones (vertebrae) and intervertebral disks. Approximately 50 irregular bones, the vertebrae are arranged in five groups: cervical (neck), thoracic (chest), lumbar (lower back), sacral (pelvic), and coccygeal (tail). The first letter of the word designating the area coupled with the number of vertebrae in the specific group constitutes the vertebral formula. (The dog is C_7, T_{13}, L_7, S_3, Cy_{20+}. The number 20 is arbitrary for the coccygeal vertebrae; many dogs have less, and a few have more.)

The intervertebral disks, elastic formations that cushion the vertebrae, allow for movement and protect against shock and related traumas. The disks absorb compression, but can't always diffuse or absorb the effects of excessive twisting or pressure on the spine.

Although the movement between any two vertebrae is limited, the vertebral column is quite flexible, except for the three sacral vertebrae, which do not have disks and are fused to form a single bone, the sacrum. All other vertebrae remain separate and move with other adjoining vertebrae in forming movable, disk-lined joints. This allows normal daily activity and maintains the necessary support.

Meninges, membranes that cover the spinal cord, are made up of three layers and protect the spinal cord from injury. The innermost layer, the pia, houses the vascular network that nourishes and removes waste from the nervous system. The arachnoid layer is the middle layer that surrounds the subarachnoid space (housing the cerebrospinal fluid). The dura mater, a protective layer on the outmost, is the strongest layer of the meninges.

Nerve fibers of each cord segment come together in the meninges to form the spinal nerves. Spinal nerves exit the spinal column between each vertebrae to innervate an area. Compression of the spinal nerves can occur with disk herniation. Inflammation and intense pain result, and affected animals exhibit lameness or hold up an affected limb. This root signature (the name given this symptom) allows the veterinarian to find the location of the compression.

DOGS AT RISK

Back problems can occur in all breeds of dogs, but there are some breeds (termed chondrodystrophic) at higher risk due to their conformation. Chondrodystrophy (faulty development of cartilage) occurs in many mammals, including humans and dogs. In humans, the condition is dwarfism, producing smaller than normal individuals whose parts are disproportionate to each other.

Some breeds of dogs, such as Dachshunds, Basset Hounds, French Bulldogs, and Corgis (both Cardigan and Pembroke), are intentionally bred (phenotypically) to produce this condition. This appearance is what draws admirers to these breeds. Although their charms are undeniable, they are at greater risk of experiencing disk abnormalities because the soft, spongy center of the disk (the nucleus pulposus) is replaced with hard cartilage. Dogs characterized by obviously short, angulated limbs are easy to identify as chondrodystrophic. However, Miniature Poodles, Beagles, Cocker Spaniels, Pekingese, Shih Tzus, and other "normal looking" dogs have been known to have chondrodystrophic disks, which occur because of the chemical makeup of the tissues of the body.

Adding to the predisposition to back injury, chondrodystrophic dogs have short legs and long backs. The movement needed for these dogs to perform everyday tasks, such as running up hills and jumping onto furniture, requires that the spine be flexed at extreme angles. These activities test flexibility, which the abnormal, hardened cartilage in the center of the disk does not allow, and heighten the possibility of rupturing disks.

SIGNS OF TROUBLE

The signs of disease can be sudden or gradual. Obviously a dog that suddenly cannot walk requires a veterinary exam, but what about the dog that occasionally stumbles or tires quickly? Should you spend the time and money to take the dog to a veterinarian? Why ask for trouble?

The intervertebral disks are elastic cushions located between each vertebra. They allow for movement and protect against shock and trauma. Understanding disease processes enlightens us to the value of recognizing early signs of disease and seeking help—thereby saving time and money in the long run and saving the dog from lingering pain and suffering.

When the owner seeks veterinary intervention, a dog's condition dictates the treatment options and their success potential. Back diseases often progress in a predictable pattern, which allows veterinarians to assess the dog's current condition and plan corrective actions.

PREDICTABILITY OF RESPONSE TO TREATMENT OF BACK DISEASE

Symptom	Treatment	Prognosis
Dog shows pain on palpation and with certain movements, but is able to walk. Pain can be intermittent or constant.	Conservative treatment begins with crate rest and limited activity. Weight reduction may be recommended, and the veterinarian may prescribe medication.	Most dogs (possibly 75%) respond with conservative treatment and return to normal activities. However, these dogs should be closely monitored for signs of disease progression.
Pet walks with unsteady or "wobbly" gait. The pet has pain or discomfort most of the time.	Confinement and rest (possibly in the animal hospital). Medication is often prescribed to relieve pain while resting. Physical therapy may be prescribed.	Conservative treatment is slightly less effective when dogs show signs of gait instability. However, it is estimated that 65% do respond at this point. Surgery may be recommended at this point, and surgical correction is very successful (95%).
Dogs are barely able to support their own weight. Pet is obviously in pain.	Absolute crate confinement is indicated. Surgery may be indicated.	Conservative treatment is successful with approximately 50% of cases; however, surgery can correct 90% of cases.

Symptom	Treatment	Prognosis
Dogs cannot support their own weight or walk on affected legs. The pet is partially or completely paralyzed, but still exhibits deep pain response.*	Surgery is recommended to relieve the pressure on the spinal cord and prevent further damage.	Only about 30% of cases will respond to conservative treatment, but 80% respond to surgical intervention.
Complete paralysis prohibits dog from moving. Dog does not exhibit deep pain response.*	Surgery is recommended to relieve severe spinal cord pressure.	Dogs do not respond to conservative treatment at this point. Surgery is only 25% effective.
Complete paralysis prohibits dog from moving. Dog exhibits continual and extreme pain. Dog does not exhibit deep pain response.*	Euthanasia due to irreparable cord bleeding.	Only 1% of dogs at this stage can be corrected, even with surgery.

*Deep pain response refers to the dog's voluntary response and awareness associated with an action (such as pinching the dog's toes) that would normally elicit pain. This response helps veterinarians determine the extent of damage to the spinal cord and thus the prognosis. The outermost fibers of the spinal cord control conscious balance and position, enabling the dog to know without looking where the four limbs, head, and tail are. The middle tracks carry fibers that control voluntary muscles and motor functions. The innermost fibers transmit involuntary actions, such as response to deep pain. When a dog does not feel deep pain, damage has penetrated through all three levels of the cord. With this extensive damage, prognosis for recovery is grave.

nts important to understand when discussing
it the pain an injured dog feels at the injury is
'n" at the injury, nor is it the same as "deep
response is tested beyond the injury. The
..s a person, a dog has a normal, involuntary
..way from pain. (i.e., pulling your hand away from
..ore your brain has even registered that it is hot is a pro-
..ex. Reflexes continue to function during most back injuries.
.eflex is absent, the prognosis worsens.)

The reflex must not be confused with a deep pain response. A positive deep pain response must be voluntary. The dog must actively pull the limb away or, if paralyzed, look at you, cry out, or try to bite in response to the pain. It must be obvious to the examiner that the dog felt the stimulus.

SPINAL CORD INJURIES

The spinal cord consists of an outer, white layer (nerve fiber tracts) and an inner, gray layer (nerve cell bodies, interconnecting fibers, and vascular supply). When injury occurs, early treatment is critical to avoid irreversible damage to the cord, which can result in permanent paralysis. If blood flow is restricted, oxygen and glucose (essential to the functioning spinal cord) cannot be delivered, and the deprived area will die. Quick surgical treatment can repair the area before permanent damage occurs. Prognosis for recovery depends on the length of time the spinal cord is deprived of adequate blood supply and the degree of injury.

Dead spinal cords liquify, at which point nothing can be done to reverse the damage. Therefore, spinal cord traumas must be treated as emergencies, and owners of injured dogs must contact their veterinarians or an emergency clinic immediately upon discovering a dog that exhibits pain and refuses to move.

Minor injuries may respond to medical management (drug therapies and crate rest). However, serious injuries require aggressive, immediate surgical intervention (preferably performed by a specialist in veterinary neurosurgery). Spinal cord trauma is most often the result of automobile accidents or disk disease and herniation.

Trauma and stress put pressure on the disks that can contribute to diseases of the back, but we cannot deny the inherited, degenerative processes of disk diseases. Understanding risks, recognizing warning signs, and securing qualified medical assistance enable dog owners to minimize the damage done to affected canine companions, thereby increasing the quality of life and the life span of their cherished pets.

INTERVERTEBRAL DISK DISEASE

Intervertebral disk disease (IVD) and herniation cause an interruption of nerve impulses in the spinal cord. This is specifically caused by a protruding or ruptured disk. This disease affects vertebrates of many species, including dogs and humans. However, the disease manifests differently in dogs than in people, partially due to the differences in posture and walking. Humans, who walk upright, are at greater risk of injury to the lumbar vertebrae, which absorb shock caused by walking and moving.

Dogs, however, walk on four legs, thus reducing the shock to the lumbar spine. Jarring forces are delivered when dogs jump or climb stairs. Force travels the length of the spinal column, sometimes causing

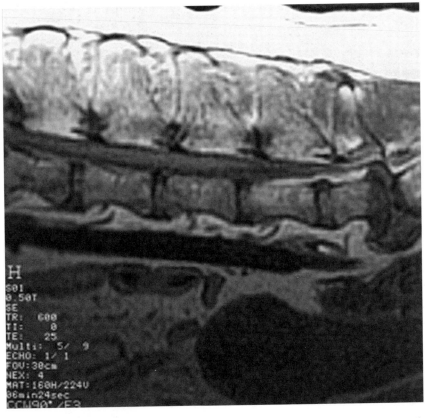

Intervertebral disk disease causes spinal cord compression due to encroachment of the misplaced disk material. Diagnosis is confirmed by either myelography or MRI. In this MRI image, the lower spinal cord is pinched in two areas (L_{6-7} and L_7-S_1).

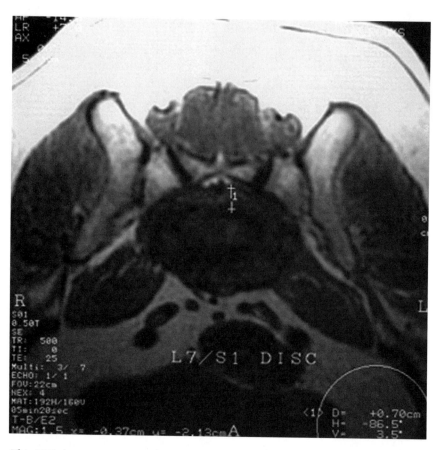

This MRI demonstrates spinal cord compression.

compression of disks and an increased risk of herniation. Herniation causes persistent, shooting pains in the legs. The signs caused by disk protrusion may vary from pain or discomfort without neurologic deficit to severe pain and paralysis or loss of muscle control from the herniated disk down.

IVD is characterized by degeneration of the disk, lessening the elasticity and flexibility. When this occurs, normal activity can cause disk displacement or rupture. The displaced disk protrudes into the spinal cord and damages the nerves. This pressure on the cord causes clinical signs of pain, weakness, or paralysis.

Due to mechanical and anatomical features in the dog, disks most often affected are in the neck and just to the rear of the last rib. Also, *humans* herniate disks *laterally,* pinching or irritating nerves as they exit the canal. *Dogs* herniate *dorsally* into the spinal cord. Rarely do humans herniate into the cord. This pressure on the cord causes clinical sig..s of pain, weakness, or paralysis.

The actual herniations caused by Hansen's type I or type II differ according to the size of the tear in the outer ring of the disk and the amount of material forced out. Although chondrodystrophic breeds make up the large majority of type I disk herniations, taxing physical activity or injury can cause this type in any mix or breed of dog.

The first type of disk degeneration (*Hansen's type I*) is seen in chondrodystrophic breeds (such as Dachshunds, Pekingese, and Shih Tzus). These dogs are characterized by short, angulated limbs. Other "normal" looking dogs have also been found to have chondrodystrophic disks, including Miniature Poodles, Cocker Spaniels, and Beagles.

Degeneration that occurs in chondrodystrophic disks occurs shortly after birth. A dramatic increase in cartilage content is seen between six and twelve months of age, reducing elasticity and shock absorption ability. Symptoms of disk herniation (in affected dogs) usually occur by two to three years of age.

The disk's soft, spongy center (nucleus pulposus) is replaced with hard cartilage. When the cartilage calcifies, the outer ring of the disk (the *annulus fibrosus*) assumes responsibility for shock absorption and, because of the added workload, begins to degenerate. This can allow it to rupture and release the thickened or calcified cartilage into the canal, thereby compressing the cord, the spinal nerves, or the nerve roots. This is disk herniation or intervertebral disk disease.

Breeds that are not chondrodystrophic are not exempt from disk herniation, however the condition rarely occurs before dogs reach

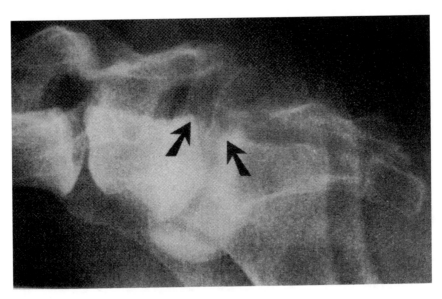

Lumbosacral instability leads to spinal misalignment and subsequent cord impingement by ossification in the spinal column.

eight years of age. This disk degeneration form of IVD usually starts at a later age (four to five years) and progresses gradually and therefore usually does not herniate until later. This condition commonly occurs in large-breed dogs.

The second type of disk degeneration (*Hansen's type II*) is the fibroid degeneration of the nucleus. This type is commonly seen in older (six to ten years old) non-chondrodystrophic breeds. The thickening starts at four to five years of age, but clinical signs are usually not apparent for many years. This is more common in large-breed dogs but may appear in any breed or mix. It progresses more slowly and generally doesn't damage the cord as severely. Medical management can sometimes control the clinical signs, but surgical intervention can be curative with no worries of future recurrence. The clinical signs usually are slow, progressive pain and weakness.

Dogs with *IVD of the neck* experience varying degrees of neck pain and stand with the head held low and the neck extended. Affected dogs resist cervical manipulation, show annoyance when the head or neck is touched, and may experience spasms of the cervical muscles. Whining and crying is common, as is a reluctance to perform routine movements.

Pain can be constant or intermittent. Rarely do cervical IVDs cause paralysis because the cervical spine has extra space in the canal, thus allowing the cord to move and not compress. Affected dogs move with stiff, short strides and may display varying degrees of a stumbling or staggering gait (tetraparesis and ataxia).

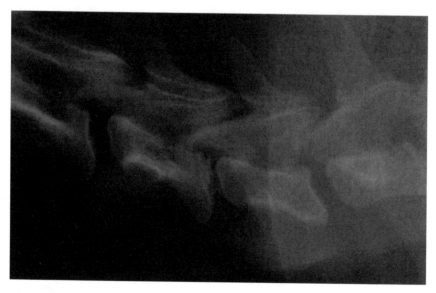

This eight-year-old, male Labrador Retriever suffers cervical IVD. Note the spinal cord compression at C_{5-6} on this myelogram due to disk rupture.

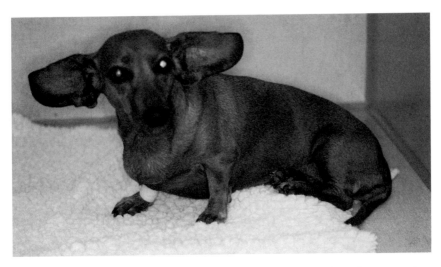

A myelogram of a seven-year-old, female Dachshund revealed cord compression due to disk rupture at T_{13}-L_1. Radiographs taken in two planes allow planning for the correct surgical approach to remove disk material.

Use of a foreleg may be restricted by a disk compressing a nerve root in the neck without causing actual spinal cord compression. The only clinical signs may be neck pain and foreleg lameness or holding up the limb, which is defined as a root signature. The location of the ruptured disk can be mapped out by a root signature.

Treatment and prognosis depend on the severity and duration of the clinical signs. Medical management with or without surgery is important to control or help reverse the inflammation and bleeding in the cord, which occurs following displacement of the disk into the cord. Surgery to relieve the pressure is usually necessary and, when indicated, should be sought immediately. The prognosis varies with each case, but if treated immediately, return to full function is usually possible, but may take two to six months and include physical therapy.

Medical management alone should be attempted on dogs with only pain or mild neurologic problems. It should also be accompanied by strict crate confinement and exercise restriction for eight to twelve weeks.

Young Great Danes and middle-aged or older Doberman Pinschers are predisposed to a cervical malformation, which can cause spinal cord compression and mimic signs of cervical IVD.

Thoracolumbar IVD disease between the last thoracic vertebra and the first lumbar vertebra is a common condition because, as the site for attachment of the last rib, there is a sudden change in stability and force between these vertebrae. Dogs with thoracolumbar IVD tend to show pain in this area, along with weakness, a stumbling or staggering gait, or paralysis of the hind limbs. The hind limb reflexes are increased. The forelimbs are normal.

Dogs with thoracolumbar IVD demonstrate a reluctance to move. An arched back may signal the presence of disease, since the dog arches to relieve pressure caused by the compressed disks. Pain (hyperesthesia) is found on manipulation of the vertebral column and is common to all IVD patients.

Lower lumbar IVD is uncommon, but when it occurs, the most common clinical signs are spinal pain, pelvic limb weakness, staggering (ataxia), paralysis, and urinary or fecal incontinence. Large-breed dogs commonly develop instability of the lumbar sacral (lumbosacral) joint, which can mimic lumbar IVD. In trying to stabilize this area, the body places bony deposits between the vertebrae, causing spinal cord compression and clinical signs like those with lower lumbar IVD.

CLINICAL SIGNS

What are the chances of a dog recovering from disk disease and returning to a good quality of life? The prognosis for treating disk disease covers a wide range. Mildly affected dogs may recover after following a prescribed period of crate rest; moderately affected dogs often require surgical intervention; and severely affected dogs occasionally receive very poor prognoses for recovery.

Without question, early detection of spinal problems is the key to obtaining the best chances for repair and recovery. Owners should carefully monitor their dogs and respond to any signs of trouble. Routine annual physical examinations by a veterinarian are especially critical for at-risk dogs. The veterinarian should assess the condition of

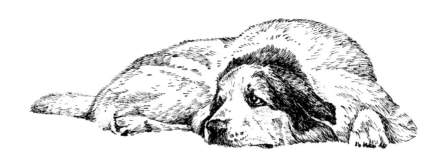

Signs of IVD vary in severity from pain without neurologic deficit to loss of motor function and pain sensation. Reluctance to walk or exercise may be your first sign that your dog needs a thorough examination.

the spine and advise the owner of the current status, likely development, and signs to watch out for and report if they occur.

The worst sign is a *lack* of pain felt when squeezing the dog's toes. Pain sensation in the limbs is most important. When this is missing for longer than 24 hours, the prognosis is grave.

DIAGNOSIS

Following physical examination, radiographs should be obtained to evaluate the condition of the spine. Radiographic signs of IVD include mineralization of the disk nucleus or annulus, narrowing or wedging of the disk space, mineralized mass within the vertebral canal, narrowing of the intervertebral opening, and collapsed facets of the vertebrae. X-rays usually appear normal or non-diagnostic because the disk is made of soft tissue, *not bone,* and therefore irregularities are not visible on radiographs unless mineralization has occurred.

If survey radiographs do not show a well-defined lesion, or if more than one lesion is found, myelography should yield additional information and would be indicated as part of the diagnostic work-up. Spinal fluid analysis may reveal cells compatible with the trauma that has occurred during disk rupture or resulting inflammation. Acute type I extrusions may show evidence of cord swelling over several vertebral bodies. The swelling is bruising and inflammation in the cord due to the sudden trauma of the disk extrusion. Type II protrusions usually are located at the front of the spinal cord. Type II disks do not cause as much trauma to the cord because of their chronic, slow course.

When available, CT scans and Magnetic Resonance Imaging (MRI) prove very useful in diagnosing IVD and differentiating it from other diseases of the spinal cord, which can cause similar symptoms. Without these diagnostic aids, neoplasia, fracture, infection, and bleeding can be confused with IVD. CT scans and MRI films provide more detailed images than myelography, but expense and availability in certain geographic areas may limit their use in veterinary medicine.

TREATMENT

Cervical IVD often can be treated with crate rest and medication. Medical management of cervical IVD is more often successful than it is with thoracolumbar or lower lumbar IVD. Because of the large canal space in the neck, IVD allows the cord to move rather than being compressed. Dogs in early stages of the disease should be confined for 14 to 21 days, and anti-inflammatory, analgesic, or muscle relaxant drugs may be prescribed. Prednisolone, aspirin, phenylbutazone, and methocarbamol often relieve symptoms of IVD with dogs under activity restriction. Pet owners often fail to follow explicit instructions to keep dogs confined and limit activity. The importance of restricting movement cannot be stressed enough, because when activity is not restricted, further injury can occur.

When recommended, surgical relief of spinal cord compression is the most effective in early stages of the disease. Decompression creates a window through the vertebral bone so that the spinal canal can be entered and examined for compressive masses or disk lesions, which can be removed.

Decompression in the neck region is usually performed from under the neck. For all other decompressive surgeries, the approach is from the top of the back.

Fenestration is another type of surgery, but is prophylactic. Fenestration can be done as a prophylatic measure to prevent degenerated disks from rupturing. Therefore, it is done before the disk ruptures. Fenestration creates an opening through which the surgeon can then remove the pulp-like body in the center of the disk, preventing disk herniation.

The procedure is somewhat controversial, and complications arise when it is performed poorly. Fenestration can be performed on surrounding disks during a decompressive surgery to prevent these disks from rupturing and compressing the cord in the future.

Postoperatively, strict exercise restriction for four to eight weeks is very important. Proper nursing care to prevent sores and urine scalding, in conjunction with physical therapy, may be necessary, depending on the patient. Bladder expression may also be necessary and can be taught to the pet owner.

Common Sites of IVD
Cervical: C_2-C_3
Thoracolumbar: T_{11}-T_{12} to L_1-L_2

CERVICAL VERTEBRAL INSTABILITY (WOBBLERS SYNDROME)

Wobblers syndrome (cervical vertebral malformation/instability syndrome) occurs in large dogs and is the result of a malformation of the vertebrae leading to disk rupture and compression of the spinal cord. A genetic predisposition is suggested, and certain breeds, including the Doberman Pinscher and the Great Dane, are at greater risk than others. The etiology of this disease remains unknown, but the high incidence seen in certain breeds suggests that heredity is a contributing factor. Overnutrition and osteochondrosis have also been cited as contributing factors.

Asymmetric growth of the cervical vertebrae causes a malformation that leads to vertebral instability or stenosis. This is usually followed by compression of the spinal cord (from the stenosis, hypertrophied soft tissue, disk rupture, or protrusion) resulting in pain and neurologic problems.

In Wobblers, the clinical signs of weakness appear most in the hind legs and without evidence of external injury. Clinical signs are usually slowly progressive (taking months or years to develop) but may occur acutely following a traumatic episode or strenuous exercise. The signs may include a reluctance to raise or lower the head (especially noticeable when called or when eating). Often an affected dog will stand with its legs set wide apart and walk with long strides causing the dog to exhibit the classic wobbling gait.

The gait may first be mildly ataxic or wobbly (hence the name) progressing to a severe, wide-based, falling stance with dragging or knuckling of the toes (walking on the top of the knuckles of the feet), mostly of the hind limbs. The forelimbs tend to appear spastic and stiff. The signs usually worsen when the dog gets up, turns, or tries to go up a stair or curb. In mild cases the condition is most evident when dogs turn corners, rather than while walking a straight line.

Older dogs (especially Dobermans and Great Danes) may become ataxic (wobbly) in the rear when they walk, while taking short, choppy steps in the front. The older dog is likely to have been experiencing difficulty getting around at home. Acutely affected dogs may be unable to stand or to lie down on their own. The dogs often appear to be arthritic, or stiff. Pressure on disks generated by the instability eventually causes degeneration and rupture of the disk. The skeletal abnormality occurs most often in the last three cervical vertebrae (five, six, and seven). Affected dogs often experience normal early lives, with symptoms taking years to appear.

Diagnosis requires an extensive evaluation of the spinal column with a myelogram, a series of radiographs performed after the injection of a contrast agent into the spinal canal that help identify the location of the lesion. Myelography is an essential aid in choosing treatment options. CT scans and MRI films help further define the disease, especially during the developmental stage before lesions become obvious.

Prescribing corticosteroids to reduce swelling may be the first treatment attempt. However, relief is usually temporary. Long-term medical management with anti-inflammatory medications, crate rest, and exercise restriction may alleviate the pain and sustain a tolerable neurologic

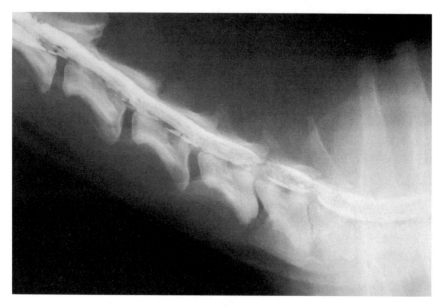

Wobblers syndrome (cervical vertebral malformation/instability) occurs in large dogs (especially in Doberman Pinschers and Great Danes). Note narrowing of the myelogram dye column at each vertebra. Compression is caused by the spinal ligament enlargement in this Doberman Pinscher.

status for some dogs for many months or even for years, but surgical repair generally enables a better recovery for the majority of cases.

Surgical correction of the instability and spinal cord compression (if present) is the long-term treatment of choice. There are two goals to surgical repair: spinal decompression and stabilization of the vertebral column. If left untreated, this disease will progress and the prognosis will be guarded in most cases.

It is important to have your dog evaluated and treated immediately if you suspect wobblers syndrome. Dogs treated in the early stages of the disease have good chances for correction and recovery; dogs treated in the later stages have more guarded prognoses. Successfully treated dogs can return to function, walk, and urinate and defecate normally without pain. However, the dogs usually continue to exhibit signs of the disease after treatment, and their gait may appear somewhat strange.

Bony changes that have already compressed the spinal cord and caused long-term damage and scarring of the cord may be irreversible. Surgery removes the compressive material and stabilizes the column, possibly allowing the cord to heal. These extreme cases are rare.

Owners electing surgical treatment for their dogs must consider the extensive nursing care required after the dog comes home from the hospital. Immediately following a myelogram or surgery, dogs often appear worse before they get better, and it can take up to two months for a pet to be able to stand without assistance.

CAUDA EQUINA/LUMBOSACRAL STENOSIS

The cauda equina is a collection of spinal roots that occupies the vertebral canal to the point of termination of the spinal cord toward the tail end. Below the sixth lumbar (L_6) vertebra, the vertebral canal has no spinal cord. Only these nerve roots are contained within the seventh lumbar (L_7) vertebra and the sacral (S) and coccygeal (C) spinal segments.

The lumbosacral spinal canal can be reduced by inflammation, trauma, or neoplasia. This reduction (stenosis) at the lumbosacral joint is called cauda equina syndrome (CES) or lumbosacral stenosis. The nerve roots become compressed, and displacement or destruction occurs. The syndrome has been associated with numerous symptoms.

Lower back pain in dogs can be attributed to the degenerative condition that compresses the nerve roots. Progressive, sharp pain is characteristic of the disease, however, dogs may be very tolerant until discomfort escalates to an intolerable level. Affected dogs experience difficulty rising and will refuse to jump. Chewing at the tail or back feet may occur as the dog attempts to relieve the burning sensation of the nerve roots, known as sciatica. Clinical signs may develop quietly, progress gradually, and present as fecal or urinary incontinence.

CES is often seen in large dogs over five years of age that have a predisposition for hip dysplasia. They frequently show lumbosacral pain, paraparesis, or lack of awareness of where a foot is placed. A history of pain during defecation is common, observed as frequent stops during the defecation process or a delay of posture after completing a bowel movement. Urinary incontinence, fecal incontinence, or tail paresis also present as problems for dogs with CES. Lameness may be intermittent.

Owners will often delay seeking treatment for their pets until painful nerve root irritation or compression has occurred. Muscle atrophy may be evident if chronic degeneration of the hind limb muscles has occurred.

Full paralysis of the hind limbs occurs in the most extreme cases of this disease. Thorough diagnostic measures must be undertaken to confirm suspicions of cauda equina syndrome. Occasionally *cauda equina* syndrome is confused with hip dysplasia if the clinical neurologic motor signs are not apparent. It is also confused with nerve root entrapment which can occur from various causes, including degenerative disk disease or tumor growth.

Stenosis at L_7-S_1 may be present, either with or without a disk protrusion. These secondary changes are believed to be caused by the instability of this joint. Large dogs have a greater incidence of this malformation, and it has been suggested that stress on the spine, due to increased body size, causes the condition.

Radiographic examination demonstrates that most patients exhibit some degree of spondylosis, with some ventral displacement or narrowing of the sacral spinal canal. Because radiographic changes must be interpreted cautiously, verification of lumbosacral disease should be done with contrast radiography (myelography), magnetic resonance imaging (MRI), CT scan, or exploratory surgery. Other causes of lumbosacral stenosis or CES may include abscesses from bite wounds or infection resulting from tail docking.

Medical treatment with corticosteroids or non-steroidal anti-inflammatory drugs (NSAIDs) may control symptoms of spinal disease initially, however, chronic progression of the disease prevents long-term management with these medications. Surgical decompression is the treatment of choice.

Veterinarians who are familiar with the technical surgical concepts of spinal surgery and understand the tissues and nerves in the area have a higher rate of success in spinal surgery. Corrective surgery is twofold—decompression of the spinal cord and stabilization of the lumbosacral vertebrae.

Proper postoperative care is essential to obtain satisfactory surgical results. Strict rest and confinement for an average of eight weeks is especially important. Owners may be required to learn the techniques of monitoring and emptying the bladder manually, as urinary control sometimes does not return for two to four weeks. Special care should be taken with the pet's bedding material to prevent decubital ulcers and/or urine burn.

Cases that have had a congenital form of stenosis diagnosed generally have a good prognosis when surgery is performed early in the course of the disease. Acquired CES or stenosis also carries a good prognosis with surgical intervention.

DEGENERATIVE MYELOPATHY (DM)

Relatively painless, slowly progressive weakening of the rear limbs is characteristic of degenerative myelopathy. Dogs may develop this condition after age five, and the condition has been reported in many breeds. However, German Shepherd Dogs and Old English Sheepdogs have reported high incidences of the disease.

Reduction of rear limb musculature and shuffling of the back legs is seen in affected dogs. Full paralysis and loss of fecal and urinary control may be present in advanced cases. Diagnosis is made following thorough neurological examination, and elevated spinal fluid protein may differentiate DM from disk disease, tumors, or other syndromes.

Treatment involves exercise, medication, and minimization of stress. Physical therapy measures and vitamin E and B therapies can sometimes revitalize DM patients. However, the stress created by major surgery (not for the DM, which cannot be treated surgically) can compromise these patients. Caution should be taken when deciding to perform surgery. Medical treatment is usually successful only in slowing or halting the progression of the disease. Uncommonly, the condition is improved. Fortunately (because there is no cure and it cannot be repaired surgically), DM is completely painless. Frustration and stress seem to be the hardest part of the disease since the animals can no longer perform as they wish. The feet also must be monitored to make sure sores don't develop once the animal becomes weak enough not to be able to pick up the feet when walking.

ATLANTOAXIAL SUBLUXATION (HYPOPLASIA OF THE DENS)

Instability or malformation of the atlantoaxial joint (the first and second cervical vertebrae) permits excessive flexion of this joint and thus compression of the spinal cord.

This can be caused by trauma in any dog, but is usually seen as a congenital or developmental malformation in Toy or Miniature breeds. Signs are usually seen within the first year of life and may have an acute onset, may be slowly progressive, or may be intermittent. The signs and onset are usually related to the activity of the dog as well as the severity of the malformation.

Clinical signs vary from reluctance to be petted on the head, to neck pain (resistance to neck movement), to weakness, or to paralysis of all four limbs. Death, due to respiratory paralysis may even occur, but is associated more frequently when trauma is the cause.

Diagnosis is made through case history, breed, physical examination, and carefully taken radiographs. The radiographs are usually taken with the dog awake (without sedation) if the animal will cooperate, because the neck muscles help protect the spinal cord by preventing the excess movement allowed by the unstable bones. Extreme care must be taken when manipulating these animals, both at home and at the animal hospital. Myelograms are usually not necessary unless spinal cord compression by other than the subluxated bones is suspected.

Animals with mild pain and no neurologic deficits or mild deficits may benefit from anti-inflammatories, a neck brace, and crate confinement for eight weeks. This may allow fibrous tissue to form and stabilize the joint. This is most successful in the smaller dogs, and repetitive therapy may be intermittently required (possibly for the rest of the pet's life) as clinical signs may recur.

Dogs with moderate to severe neurologic deficits or pain, or dogs unresponsive to medical management, should undergo surgery to stabilize the joint. Usually pins, wires, and/or bone grafts are used to stabilize the area. This is a dynamic disease where compression occurs with movement, but permanent or secondary compressive lesions do not usually appear with this disease.

Prognosis is fair to good, unless acute paralysis of all four limbs occurs, which may indicate severe cord trauma. The instability can be corrected, but the severe trauma can irreversibly damage the cord. If atlantoaxial subluxation is suspected, exercise and manipulation must be kept to a minimum until the dog can be evaluated by a veterinarian.

FIBROCARTILAGENOUS EMBOLUS

Fibrocartilagenous embolus is generally seen in large-breed dogs of any age. The clinical signs of neurologic deficits can vary depending on where the lesion is, but the signs are usually obviously asymmetrical. Diagnosis is usually made by appropriate history and a physical and neurologic exam. All tests such as plain radiography and myelography are usually normal and thus other causes are ruled out.

This is a disease in which an embolus occludes an artery or vein of the spinal cord, causing necrosis in that area. Origin of the embolus is unknown. The disease is characterized by an acute onset of neurologic deficits. It is usually not painful and nonprogressive (after the first few hours). Although the relationship is unknown, some dogs with this disease have a history of mild to moderate exercise or minor trauma prior to the onset of clinical signs. Many have nothing unusual in their histories.

The basis of treatment is good nursing care, physical therapy, and time. Anti-inflammatories may help in the beginning, but after several days they are usually no longer beneficial. Clinical improvement generally occurs within two weeks, but it may take months to recover fully. Due to the location of some lesions, dogs can suffer irreversible spinal cord damage and thus have a poor prognosis for a return to function.

CHAPTER 11

OTHER CAUSES
OF LAMENESS

Lameness can be caused by sources not usually considered when one thinks about the skeletal structure. Occasionally, a dog's inability to walk or stand is the first observable indicator of underlying disease.

In addition to malformation of bones, metabolic disease, neoplasia, and neurological problems can manifest themselves as orthopedic diseases. Understanding their impact and influences on the musculoskeletal system aids in the diagnosis, treatment, and care of the canine orthopedic patient. The physical examination should include evaluation of the spine and a series of laboratory tests when indicated.

The presence of spinal pain suggests spinal lesions. In such cases direct palpation of the vertebra will elicit a painful response. When a neurologic cause of lameness is suspected, the veterinarian will evaluate each section of the vertebrae to assess pain response. Pain when pressure is placed on the bone at the base of the neck may indicate damage to the cervical region of the spine. Similarly, pressure to the muscles slightly below the ribs (epaxial) that elicits pain suggests damage to the thoracolumbar region.

Orthopedic problems related to the physical and chemical function of internal organs that build and maintain the animal's living system are related to the metabolism. Of particular interest are the endocrine glands, which secrete hormones and have a regulatory effect on the skeletal structure. Nutritional imbalances can be involved in this group of orthopedic problems. Metabolic disease can also cause weakness that may seem to be an orthopedic or neurological problem, but in reality may be something else.

Metabolic bone disease can include a variety of conditions that develop into a secondary reduction of bone mass known as osteopenia, an imbalance in bone formation and resorption. Frequently, the animal exhibits signs of the primary disease, with the musculoskeletal symptoms being less obvious.

METABOLIC OSTEOPENIA

Endocrine disorders can include increased or decreased activity of the parathyroid or adrenal glands, common metabolic diseases. These glands can alter the metabolism of bone, causing osteoporosis, stress fractures, and weakened ligaments.

Hyperparathyroidism, an abnormal increase in the production of parathyroid hormone, robs the bones of calcium. These bones become weak and brittle and are easily broken. Parathyroid hormone is normally released in response to low blood calcium and maintains a normal blood calcium/phosphorus ratio. However, in diseased dogs, the mineral balance is askew and affects the dogs' ability to efficiently support their body systems.

There are two types of hyperparathyroidism—primary and secondary *Primary hyperparathyroidism* prevents placement of calcium in the blood to the teeth and bones, causing those structures to become weak and break. The condition is caused by a benign (not cancerous) tumor that grows on one or more of the four parathyroid glands. The condition can be present in dogs, yet undetected until the symptoms of breaking bones or kidney disease (caused from processing excess calcium from the blood through the kidneys) manifest. Primary hyperparathyroidism occurs in older dogs, usually more than eight years of age.

Primary hyperparathyroidism should be suspected when blood tests display elevated calcium, and other causes (neoplasias) have not been detected. Any dog can develop the condition, which has often been seen in Keeshonden, Samoyeds, Salukis, Papillons, and mixed-breed dogs.

Surgical removal of the diseased, hyperactive parathyroid, followed by intensive post-operative care, yields good prognoses for a return to active life. However, extreme caution should be taken when selecting a surgeon and a critical care supportive hospital. Dogs typically experience extreme drops in calcium blood levels at day four following surgery. This life threatening situation often requires IV administration of calcium and close monitoring of calcium levels to sustain the patient.

Therapies include injectable and oral administration of calcium, vitamin D, and magnesium until the previously suppressed remaining parathyroid glands are strong enough to support the patient. Owners should be cautioned to observe their pets for signs of calcium depletion throughout the pet's life. Panting, seizures, muscle twitching, a wobbling gait, elevated temperature, staring, and cramping pains signal the need for immediate veterinary examination.

Secondary renal hyperparathyroidism (renal osteodystrophy) can also compromise bone health. The clinical signs of renal disease will often be dominant; however, young, growing dogs with congenital

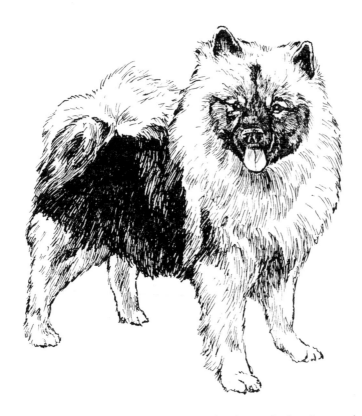

Owners of purebred dogs should become familiar with the diseases known to occur in their breeds. For example, primary hyperparathyroidism causes bone degeneration and can affect Keeshonden. Blood tests can screen for the disease (which usually occurs at about eight years of age), making treatment possible.

Illustration by Chris Hoy

renal disease may demonstrate more obvious signs of bone disease, such as lameness, pain, and spontaneous fractures. The skeletal lesions are related to the amount of excess parathyroid hormone that has been produced, as well as the length of time the condition has been on-going and the age of the dog.

Skeletal changes may be first and most apparent in the structure of the head, seen as the pliable "rubber jaw" or loosened teeth. Treatment is focused on the primary renal disease process, and cage rest is enforced to prevent skeletal damage or fracture. Dietary changes are made to control protein intake, for the kidney disease, and to possibly supplement dietary calcium.

Nutritional secondary hyperparathyroidism can result from a diet low in calcium, high in phosphorus, or deficient in vitamin D. An all-meat diet, for example, lacks the nutrient balance found in commercial dog foods. Secondary hyperparathyroidism may also be caused by gastrointestinal malabsorption of calcium or glucocorticoid excesses. Gastrointestinal malabsorption can be caused by agents that bind calcium in the GI tract, preventing absorption. Something as seemingly benign as mineral oil has been implicated as such an agent. Treatment is based on correcting the diet and guarding against fractures during the rehabilitation period.

Hyperadrenocorticism can also cause osteopenia. Also known as Cushing's disease, this condition can occur in middle-aged or older dogs, with some increase in breed incidence noted in Poodles, Dachshunds, Boston Terriers, and Boxers. With this condition, the outer layer (cortex) of the adrenal gland produces excess glucocorticoids. This can be caused by a tumor involving the adrenal gland or a tumor of the pituitary that regulates the adrenal gland. Cushing's can also be caused by excessive steroid medication.

Myasthenia gravis (MG) affects the interaction of nerves and muscles. The disease can be congenital or acquired, and large breeds are most frequently affected. Dogs with MG exhibit muscle weakness, with congenital cases becoming obvious by eight weeks of age when puppies learn to walk and move about. Acquired forms are most often associated with a benign tumor of the thymus gland.

Dogs with MG tire easily during exercise, but recover after a short rest. Dogs may shorten their strides to conserve energy, may show discomfort in their facial expression, and may lower the head while walking, standing, or sitting. An enlarged esophagus (megaesophagus) can accompany the disease, and pneumonia may result from undigested foods, which are regurgitated and aspirated.

The most commonly used diagnostic test for MG is the Edrophonium chloride (Tensilon) response test. Dogs are injected with this substance, and an improvement in muscle stability seen within 30 seconds and lost within five minutes may confirm suspicions of MG. Prostigmin may be substituted for Tensilon, or radiographs of the chest may be utilized to detect tumors of the thymus or esophagus enlargement.

Treatment for MG in the dog includes use of anticholinesterase drugs and removal of the thymus when tumors are present. Pyridostigmine bromide (Mestinon) is the current drug of choice for acquired MG, and Neostigmine (Prostigmin) has also been used. Veterinarians must medicate MG dogs cautiously. Some antibiotics, heart medications, and other drugs can increase the symptoms of MG in the dog.

Meningitis, an inflammatory disease of the brain covering (meninges) is usually a result of infection (bacterial or fungal). The disease can occur in any breed or any age dog, but young dogs (under 18 months of age)

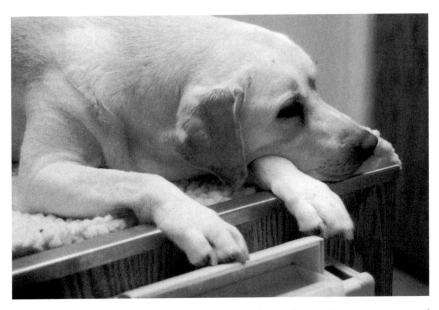

A dog's reluctance to exercise can signify underlying disease. Report any unusual changes in activity to your veterinarian, who may recommend tests to uncover the reason for the apathy.   *Photo by Leslie Bird*

are the usual victims. Meningitis causes weakness, seizures, dementia, neck pain, and other clinical signs. Diagnosis requires examination of the cerebrospinal fluid, which may exhibit increased white blood cell counts, increased protein, and elevated pressures. The treatment of choice involves antibiotics or antifungals, according to the specific bacteria or fungus present.

Cancer is an uncontrolled growth of cells on or within the body. It can be localized, or it can invade adjacent tissue and spread (metastasize) throughout the body. Various forms of cancer affect the orthopedic status of animals. Cancer is common in pets, and the risk increases with age. Dogs get cancer at roughly the same rate as humans, and, according to the American Veterinary Medical Association, pet owners should be aware of the common signs of cancer in small animals:

- Abnormal swellings that persist or continue to grow

- Sores that do not heal

- Weight loss

- Loss of appetite

- Bleeding or discharge from any body opening

- Offensive odor

- Difficulty eating or swallowing

- Hesitation to exercise or loss of stamina

- Persistent lameness or stiffness

- Difficulty breathing, urinating, or defecating

Hypertrophic Osteopathy is a condition that occurs secondarily with a thoracic mass (or less frequently an abdominal mass) of metastatic or localized nature. Geriatric patients are most commonly affected by this condition. It is believed to be caused by an increased blood flow to the extremities. The increase in circulation can cause swelling of all four limbs, first at the farthest point, then progressing closer to the trunk of the dog's body. The joints are not usually involved.

Clinical signs include pain and lameness of all four limbs. Treatment for hypertrophic osteopathy includes surgical removal of the mass, or a lobectomy or pulmonectomy of an affected lung. The clinical signs will retreat after corrective surgery; however, prognosis usually is guarded due to the underlying cancer. Infrequently, other non-neoplastic conditions may cause hypertrophic osteopathy, usually diseases related to the lungs.

NEOPLASIA

Bone weakness can occasionally be attributed to underlying disease, such as cancer. Depending on the type, location, and localization of each tumor, treatment may include surgery, chemotherapy, and/or radiation. Many cancers are controllable, and a veterinary oncologist is best prepared to diagnose and treat cancer. Thanks to technological advances seen in veterinary medicine, cancer is no longer unbeatable.

Skeletal neoplasia (cancer) is almost always malignant. There is a high occurrence of neoplastic bone disease in dogs, and it often develops rapidly.

There have been many improvements in the treatment of cancer in the last decade. Surgical amputation, or limb sparing when combined with chemotherapy, can extend the dog's life. Limb-sparing surgery involves tumor removal and limb reconstruction using bone grafts and plates. Complications can include local tumor recurrence and infection.

Chemotherapy (treatment of cancer through the use of medication) is often used in combination with amputation or limb-sparing surgery. These therapies may also be combined with radiation therapy for prolonged survival times. When suspecting a bone cancer, radiographic

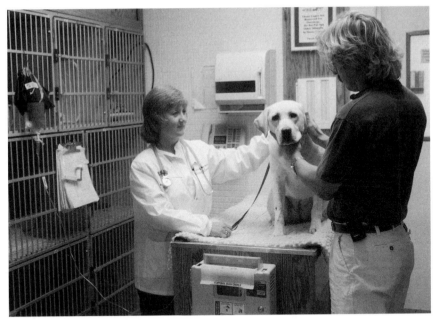

Many cancers affect the bones. However, most can be treated with surgery, chemotherapy, and/or radiation.   *Photo by Leslie Bird*

evaluation of the affected limb, as well as three views of the chest, should be taken. Additional x-rays screen for metastases in the chest, which can be common with primary bone cancer.

When chemotherapy is recommended as part of the treatment protocol, a thorough evaluation of blood chemistries and a complete blood cell count should be performed prior to (and periodically during) the chemotherapy.

Osteosarcoma is the most common primary bone tumor in dogs. It is frequently found in middle-aged and older dogs of large breeds. The causes of osteosarcoma have not been identified, however, the most common sites include the radius, humerus, femur, and tibia.

Smaller dogs tend to have a greater proportion of axial skeletal neoplasias than those located in the extremities. A definite diagnosis of osteosarcoma must be made with a biopsy of the affected area of bone. Signs of osteosarcoma are lameness, pain, and/or a local swelling of the extremity.

Chondrosarcomas are the second most common bone tumors found in dogs. Affecting mostly large dogs, chondrosarcomas usually affect flat bones, such as the ribs and pelvis. In later stages the tumor can metastasize to the lungs. Usually occurring as a primary tumor, chondrosarcomas grow more slowly than osteosarcomas and generally

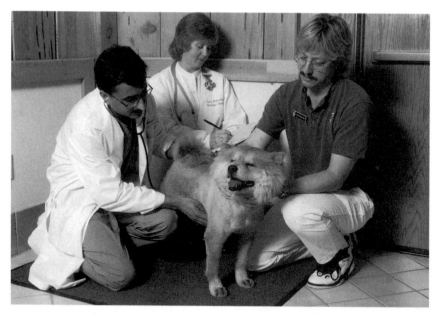

Cancer patients should receive regular, thorough examinations. This Chow Chow is being treated for osteoscarcoma and still enjoys good quality of life.

Photo by Leslie Bird

have a longer course of disease. Although the tumor can be removed surgically, the chance of local recurrence is a concern.

Fibrosarcomas occur in the medium- and large-breed dogs, with males more commonly affected than females. Fibrosarcoma primary tumors are rare, but they may recur at a surgery site if amputation or limb-sparing surgery is not used with chemotherapy (cisplatin). *Hemangiosarcomas,* which occur as primary bone tumors, are rare. Affecting medium and large dogs, the clinical signs include lameness, localized swelling, and pain.

Metastases can occur in the lungs, spleen, liver, and right atrium. Because of the possibility of metastasis, a thorough evaluation should be made utilizing abdominal ultrasound and chest x-rays. In some cases a nuclear bone scan is indicated to check for multiple skeletal tumors.

Bone cysts can occur in young, large-breed dogs. The Doberman Pinscher and German Shepherd Dog have been identified most frequently with this skeletal disease. Usually, bone cysts are found in one site; however, multiple cysts occur in some cases.

The cystic cavity is filled with a blood-tinged fluid. If there is suspicion of neoplasia, aspiration of the cystic cavity is suggested. If lameness is the result of a bone cyst, surgical drainage, curettage, and/or a bone graft may be appropriate therapies.

FUNGAL OSTEOMYELITIS

Disseminated musculoskeletal fungal infections can occur with many of the fungal organisms, including coccidiomycosis, blastomycosis, histoplasmosis, cryptococcosis, and aspergillosis. More animals are becoming susceptible to mycotic infection due to veterinary advanced skin cancer chemotherapy, organ transplantation, broad spectrum antibiotics, and immunosupressive medications.

Fungal lesions may be singular or multiple. Diagnosis of fungal disease should be made by blood tests, radiography, and biopsy of the lesions. Fungal osteomyelitis is treated with antifungal drugs. Long-term therapy regimens are often necessary for control of the organism.

Diagnostic tests to uncover the reason for lameness may include blood tests, biopsies, and/or a variety of x-rays.

Photo by Leslie Bird

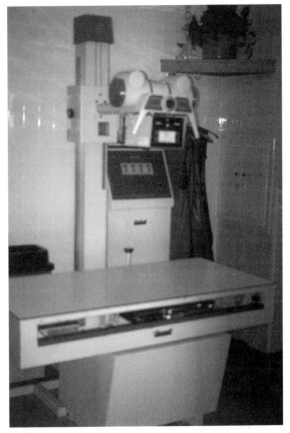

DEGENERATIVE MYELOPATHY (DM)

A painless, progressive weakening of the rear limbs is characteristic of *degenerative myelopathy*. Dogs may develop this condition after age five, and the condition has been reported in many breeds. However, German Shepherd Dogs and Old English Sheepdogs have reported high incidences of the disease.

Reduction of rear limb musculature and shuffling of the back legs is seen in affected dogs. Full paralysis and loss of fecal and urinary control may appear in advanced cases. Diagnosis is made following a thorough neurological examination, and elevated spinal fluid protein may differentiate DM from disk disease, tumors, or other syndromes.

Treatment involves exercise, medication, and reduction of stress. Physical therapy measures and vitamin E and B therapies can revitalize DM patients. However, stress created by major surgery for conditions other than DM can compromise these patients. Caution should be taken when making the decision to perform surgery on them.

CHAPTER 12

TRAUMA-INDUCED ORTHOPEDIC DISEASE— ACCIDENT PREVENTION AND FIRST AID

Too many pets and pet owners are familiar with the pain associated with traumatic accidents. Veterinary emergency hospitals consider car accident victims common occurrences, and other bodily injuries present themselves daily. The owners of injured dogs tell of their pets being hit by a golf club (a Pomeranian tried to steal the ball as the owner was teeing up), falling from a balcony (especially common in urban settings), and being knocked against the wall while wrestling with another dog.

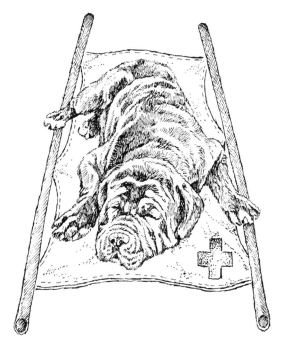

Quick response to an accident is often needed in order to save a life or a limb.
Illustration by Chris Hoy

BLONDIE'S STORY

Blondie, a lovely Afghan Hound, was picked up by animal control last summer. She had been running in the streets and was hit by a car. Blondie waited in a kennel (under sedation) for three days, while humane society owners hoped her owners would appear to claim her, but they never showed. After three days Blondie became property of the humane society, and they considered aggressive treatment to repair her fractured pelvis. Unfortunately, Blondie's injuries were quite extensive; her pelvis was fractured in four locations, so healing would be a lengthy process. Trauma-related orthopedic injuries are perhaps the most easily prevented musculoskeletal problems seen in dogs. However, nobody thinks accidents will happen to them. Only hindsight is 20/20.

Not all traumatic injuries present life-or-death situations. The major consequences resulting from injury range in severity and include inflammation, loss of function, and infection. Minor injuries can be treated at home, using homeopathic remedies or over-the-counter medications. However, most injuries should be seen by a veterinarian to determine the extent of damage. Some internal injuries are not visible.

The veterinarian will assess not only the external injuries, but will consider internal damage as well. Often the "hidden" traumas present the greatest long-term threats to afflicted dogs. Adjacent tissues or organs can be damaged from trauma associated with fractures. Radiographic evaluation from at least two views is needed to determine the diagnosis, the prognosis, and the best method of treatment.

Trauma is a wound or injury inflicted suddenly by a physical action to the body and often occurs when proper methods of restraint are ignored. Traumatic injuries occur in urban and suburban areas and can be fatal if left untreated. Urban areas have high incidences of trauma cases caused by sharp objects (metal and glass on the ground) and falls from great heights. Rural dogs have an increased incidence of injuries caused by weapons (primarily firearms). Young animals are more commonly involved in traumatic incidents.

Injuries to dogs often result from motor vehicle accidents (54%) and interaction with other animals (11%). Unknown causes account for approximately 12% of traumatic injuries to pets. The extremities (legs and feet) receive the highest proportion of injuries (45%), and the severity of the injuries vary from minor to moderate, with a small percentage considered life threatening.

ACCIDENT PREVENTION

All would agree that an ounce of prevention *is* worth a pound of cure. But even cautious dog owners can experience the pain of having their pets injured in "freak" accidents. However, precautionary measures can be taken to minimize the risks to our cherished family members.

Start by looking at the world from your dog's eyes. What dangers do you see?

IN THE HOME

Consider the size, age, and temperament of your dog. Get on your knees and assess the environment. Owners of small dogs should be aware of boxes and other items that could fall. Puppy owners should guard their pups from the dangers of falling through slats in a staircase. Older dogs can be harmed by falls on a slick floor. Identify threats to your dog's safety, and fix the situation.

OUTDOORS

The leash is your friend. Too many owners jeopardize their dogs by giving them too much freedom. Even well-trained dogs can become distracted by cats, noises, rabbits, or movements and can take off without thinking, falling victim to moving traffic.

SECURE YOUR YARD

Consider access areas and your dogs' capability of expanding or creating their own exits. Put locks on gates (and use them) to prohibit accidental escapes from gates left ajar. Safely store gardening and construction equipment. Be sure traffic areas are free of foot-catching hazards.

SPAY AND NEUTER YOUR PETS

The mating urge can motivate normally placid pets to complete Herculean feats. Intact males often jump fences to get to a bitch in heat, only to meet up with accidents. Bitches in heat sometimes display the same tendencies and are at risk of injury.

TRAUMA BASICS

Trauma is caused by variables within the environment (strain) or by forces generated within the animal (stress). Three kinds of stress/strain cause traumatic injury when delivered with unnatural strength, length, or onset: tension, compression, and shearing. *Tension* is produced when a structure is pulled apart or elongated. *Compression* is the result of being pushed together or shortened. *Shear force* occurs when the object resists a sliding action.

The mass (body size) of the animal influences the degree of injury incurred with any stress or strain, and the length of time that the stress

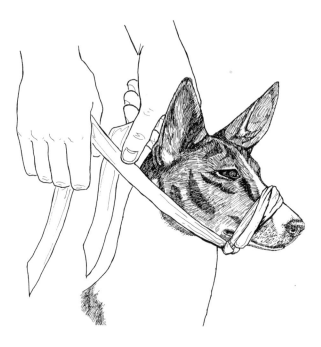

Injured dogs often exhibit aggression. Securely muzzle any dog that may bite during transport or treatment.   *Illustration by Monique Raymond*

or strain is applied impacts the degree of traumatic injury, with the longer exposure generating greater damage to tissues and bone. Athletes know the damage done when they fail to properly warm up before beginning strenuous exercise, so do dogs.

Simple rules of physics tell us that larger surface areas of contact absorb force better, resulting in injury reduction. Considering dogs, the same amount of force impacting a Great Dane and a Chihuahua will have a less severe effect on the Great Dane.

Owners of fragile dogs should be especially aware of the chance of injury. Observe small dogs carefully for lameness or discomfort, possibly caused by unnoticed daily activities. For instance, some lightly built Toy breeds frequently fracture their front legs (radius/ulna) by jumping. Their bones are so fragile that the force on impact is too severe for absorption of the force.

INFLAMMATION

Synovitis is the inflammation of the soft tissue of the joint and the synovial membrane that lines the joint cavity. The synovial membrane is important to the normal functioning of a joint, and inflammation leads to thickening of the capsule, which can interfere with range of motion of the joint and cause pain.

Athletic animals suffer most frequently from joint inflammation. Training and competition often place stress and strain on the joint greater than the forces the joint was designed to withstand. The result is a stretching of the joint capsule and inflammation of the soft tissue. This leads to heat, pain, swelling, reduced range of motion, and lameness. Early recognition of synovitis, along with the proper therapy, can stop, or even reverse, these events.

When the synovial membrane becomes inflamed from trauma or injury, the consequences are almost immediate. The blood vessels near the membrane dilate, and the walls of the vessels leak fluid and cells into the joint cavity, causing swelling and pain. If synovitis is not treated and the joint stress continues, the inflammatory response attacks and damages the articular cartilage. The damaged cartilage will no longer have the cushioning effect and the shock absorption ability on the joint.

The forces that once were normal are now altered and create a cycle of damage and degeneration. Once damage to bone begins, it can be seen on x-rays. However, by the time you can detect this process on film, permanent damage has occurred, and the joint can never be fully restored to normal.

MUSCLE INJURIES

Muscle injuries are very common in athletic dogs. While these injuries are occasionally dramatic and cause severe pain and lameness, they are frequently more subtle and may cause few signs other than a sub-par performance or reluctance to perform.

Bruising (contusion) of the muscle, a very common injury, is frequently associated with the tearing of muscle fibers, a condition known as muscle strain. The clinical signs of bruising (swelling, heat, localized pain, and discoloration of the skin) may or may not be obvious. Lameness can occur, depending on the location of the injury.

These injuries can be pinpointed by careful palpation. Pain and muscle spasms (twitching) should be evident when the area is palpated. In active dogs, these injuries commonly occur in the muscles of the neck, back, and shoulders.

Rupture (tearing) of the tendon attached to a specific muscle occurs from stress, a sharp blow, a deep laceration, a fall, or a gunshot wound. Some breeds show a high tendency to develop such injuries, which may indicate a genetic predisposition for tendon rupture. Animals subjected to more work or exercise than their muscles are prepared to do suffer muscle fatigue and are prone to injury. An exhausted dog may overextend or overflex muscles and may not be able to compensate for sudden changes in terrain or ground surface. The tendon frequently tears before the muscle.

Ligament injury, often associated with fatigue, can include strains and sprains, tears, or detachment. Ligament damage can include elbow luxation, carpal sprain, and stifle injuries.

The ligament has minimal elasticity, and when the fibers of the ligament become elongated by 10% or more, damage occurs. When a ligament becomes damaged, the affected joint becomes unstable and function is lost. Surgical repair of the ligament is generally required to restore function. Nonsurgical treatment may leave the joint unstable, resulting in chronic degenerative joint disease and lameness.

Loss of Function

Fractures come to mind when considering possible causes of loss of function. A fracture, or a break in the bone, can range in severity from a small fissure, a greenstick fracture, or a complete, displaced fracture. Treatment of fractured bones varies with location and type of fracture. However, normal healing is most often the result, with return to normal or near normal function.

A *fissure fracture* consists of one or more small cracks penetrating the outer layer of the bone (cortex). The *greenstick fracture* involves

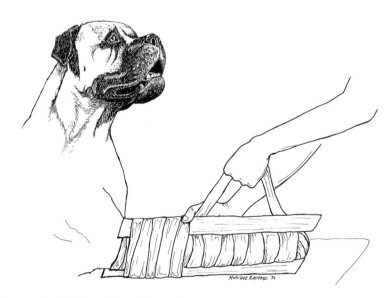

A fracture that is below the stifle or elbow can be splinted by using a rolled magazine, newspaper, or clothes hanger for support, secured with materials found at home, such as nylons, belts, ties, or duct tape. *Illustration by Monique Raymond*

a fracture in one side of the bone with the other side bent, and it occurs primarily in young, growing dogs. A *complete fracture* is a total disruption of the bone, (both cortexes are fractured) with abnormal positioning of the fragments.

Fractures can occur in a multitude of directions within the bone, including transverse, oblique, and spiral. The location of a fracture may involve a fragment of bone (avulsion) detached with a portion of muscle, tendon, or ligament.

Physeal fractures occur in young, growing dogs in growth plate areas. The rounded ends of the bones (condyles) may be separated from the portion of the long bone either singularly or may involve both condyles, creating three or more fragments. The fracture site can be *closed,* with no outside wound associated with the fractured portions of bone, or open. *Open fractures* in which bone segments penetrate through the skin are highly susceptible to infection, complicating the healing process.

CAUSES OF FRACTURES

Bone fractures are often caused by trauma from direct or indirect force. Environmental conditions often contribute to fracture. Pathologic Fractures occur when for example nutritional or neoplastic diseases weaken bone, predisposing it to fracture from daily activity or otherwise minor trauma. Repeated stress can cause fractures from fatigue in performance dogs.

Fractures occur less frequently to the forelimb than to the hind limb, perhaps due to the flexible nature of the muscular forelimb support. The hind limbs are rigidly joined with the rest of the skeleton, increasing the incidence of fracture. Pelvic fractures are involved in approximately 30% of all fractures in dogs, mostly associated with motor vehicle accidents.

Every fracture can be treated with various methods, and the personal preferences of the practitioner may influence the route chosen. The amount of weight carried by the forelimbs increases the need for a rigid setting of forelimb fractures. Complicated fractures require the attention of highly skilled surgeons. Referral to a specialist is often indicated. This is especially important because fractures repaired correctly will heal quickly and normally, whereas incorrect repair of a fracture may cause deformed healing, joint problems, or failure to heal at all (nonunion).

DISLOCATION/LUXATION

Disruption of normal joint anatomy is described as a dislocation or luxation. When luxation occurs, surrounding synovial joint structures may

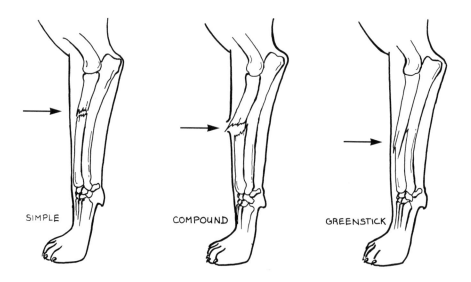

SIMPLE   COMPOUND   GREENSTICK

Broken bones vary in severity of fracture and in treatment requirements.

become damaged, and ligament damage usually accompanies dislocation of a joint. Complete luxation of a joint occurs when the bones
are severely displaced and have no continuity. Damage to the joint ligaments becomes serious, and immediate, appropriate stabilization is
necessary for the best recovery outcome.

Trauma is the most common cause of luxation, and various joints
of the forelimb can be affected. Elbow dislocations occur most frequently, and shoulder dislocations are occasionally seen in dogs.
Carpal joint dislocations are frequent injuries resulting from accidents.
The hip (coxofemoral) joint is the most frequent luxation of all dog
joints, *and although hip dysplasia can develop into luxation, trauma is
the most common cause for dislocation of the hip.*

Although singular ligament rupture involving the cruciate ligament
is extremely frequent, stifle dislocation is rarely seen in dogs. Athletic,
older, and obese dogs can experience tarsal subluxation or dislocation
from running or jumping movements. Shear injuries and severe trauma
are additional causes of tarsal dislocation.

INFECTION

The skin acts as a natural barrier to infection and contamination.
Trauma from mechanical injury often results in destruction of membranes. Underlying tissue spaces are thereby exposed and open to
contamination from bacteria and foreign materials. If contamination is

extensive, or with cases involving large amounts of tissue destruction, the possibility of infection can become overwhelming.

Infection is not usually an immediate occurrence; however, the threat of infection becomes a vital concern in the management and treatment of any orthopedic injury, especially an open fracture. Invasive infection further destroys tissue, causing loss of function and possible septic conditions. Septic shock can result 48 hours or more following the injury, and death can ensue.

Osteomyelitis, infection in a bone, may result in bone destruction or the stiffening of joints, depending on the extent of infection. Factors influencing infection of fracture repair sites include the type of bone, whether the fracture was open or closed, and the extent of soft tissue damage. Animals with contaminated wounds are more likely to develop infections or experience complications in fracture healing. Immediate flushing of a contaminated wound with warm water can reduce the amount of infection.

FIRST AID/TRANSPORTATION

What should you do if your dog is injured? Immediate care of the traumatized dog begins at home, and appropriate action on the part of the

Pins can be implanted to stabilize broken bones. When properly treated, injured dogs can return to full function.

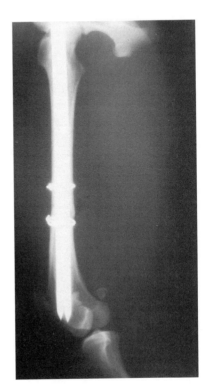

owner can prevent further injury to an animal. However, pet owners should be cautious to avoid injuries to themselves, resulting from attempts to help an injured pet, because even the sweetest animals suffering pain may bite.

Dog owners should familiarize themselves with the principles of CPR. Clearing an airway is the first priority in first aid treatment. Blood loss is another serious concern. Stop bleeding as soon as possible by applying direct pressure to the area around bleeding wounds.

Prepare the injured dog for transport. A fracture that is below the stifle or elbow can be splinted by using a rolled magazine, newspaper, or clothes hanger for support, secured with materials found at home, such as nylons, belts, ties, or duct tape. Fractures above this point cannot be immobilized without potentially causing more damage by adding a fulcrum point.

Visible penetrating foreign bodies should not be removed but should be stabilized during transportation to the veterinary hospital. Removing objects from body cavities or limbs may result in additional bleeding or damage to the soft tissue structure. Transportation on a stiff board is recommended until complete evaluation of injuries can be performed at the veterinary hospital. Orthopedic injuries, especially those associated with open fractures, are considered serious conditions and require immediate veterinary emergency care.

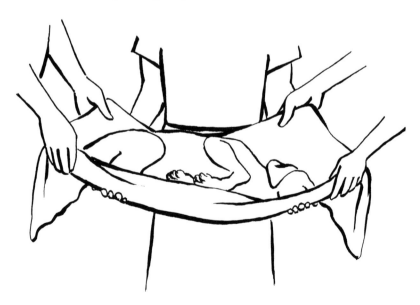

Take care in transporting injured dogs. Stabilize any possible fractures and use a board or blanket to carry the dog.   *Illustration by Monique Raymond*

TREATMENTS

CHAPTER 13

NATURE OR NURTURE?
ENVIRONMENTAL INFLUENCES ON ORTHOPEDIC AND NEUROLOGICAL DISEASE

The goal in dealing with any disease is, of course, prevention. In dealing with orthopedic diseases, much discussion has been given to the debate of nature vs. nurture in the cause of growth-related lameness, and especially in regard to hip dysplasia. It is generally accepted that genetics contributes to orthopedic diseases, but that environmental influences contribute to the likelihood or variability of expression of the various diseases.

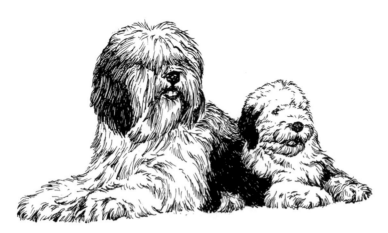

Fast-growing, large dogs are especially affected by dietary influence.

Illustration by Chris Hoy

Factors other than inheritance affect the development of hip dysplasia and other orthopedic diseases. Environmental factors, such as nutrition and exercise, can have considerable influence as well. Factors inherent to the dog also have an influence, such as pelvic muscle mass, excessive estrogens (the normal biological range will not cause it), and rapid growth.

DIET AND ORTHOPEDIC DISEASE

Nutrition does have an influence on hip dysplasia. The primary influential factor lies in a high-protein diet that will cause rapid growth. By limiting the protein, one can prevent abnormally rapid growth and lessen the incidence or severity of the disease without stunting the dog's growth. Puppies will grow to their potential size, just at a slower rate.

Because nutrition influences every aspect of a dog's health and fitness, generalizations about what to feed them should be avoided. Veterinarians should counsel their clients by taking into consideration the size, age, and general health of the individual dog. However, experts recommend feeding an amount of dietary protein at about 21% to 24% for most dogs.

Hip dysplasia is a polygenic disease, meaning that it is influenced by many genes as well as many external factors. Hereditary influence

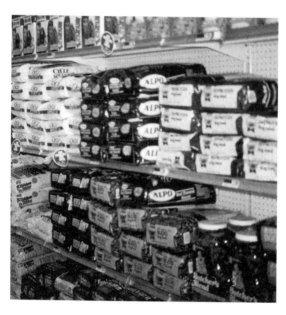

Read the labels on dog food bags. High amounts of calcium, protein, or calories may increase a puppy's chances of developing degenerative joint disease.

cannot be ignored, but *diets high in protein, calories, and calcium can encourage the expression of hip dysplasia.* Therefore, fast-growing large dogs are especially affected by dietary influence. Very young puppies may be fed higher amounts of protein, but the protein amount should be restricted to 21 to 24% at four months of age in large breeds and six months in medium and small breeds. Feeding young, growing puppies a particular food type or supplement to encourage maximum growth rates will increase the risk of all skeletal diseases.

According to an article that appeared in the *Journal of the American Veterinary Medical Association,* trial feeding of Labrador Retriever puppies supports the theory of dietary influence: *"Restricting the food consumption of growing Labrador Retrievers to 24% less food than their ad libitum pair-fed littermates resulted in a marked reduction in the expression of hip dysplasia."*

Twenty-four pairs of littermates were evaluated from the time they were eight weeks old until they were two years old. Hip joints when the dogs were two years old were evaluated on radiographs by use of the standard position (limbs extended) and scored according to the Orthopedic Foundation for Animals method and the Swedish scoring method.

> *"The incidence of hip dysplasia was 25% in the limit-fed group, whereas the incidence was 71% in the ad libitum-fed group. It is concluded that these data supported the clinical recommendations to avoid overfeeding growing dogs, particularly those breeds prone to hip dysplasia, and substantiated earlier observations that limiting food intake was beneficial in preventing the expression of hip dysplasia."*

Source: "Effects of Limited Food Consumption on the Incidence of Hip Dysplasia in Growing Dogs," *JAVMA* 1992, 201:6. 857-63; 28 ref. Kealy, R.D., Olsson, S.E., Monti, K.L., Lawler, D.F., Biery, D.N., Helms, R.W., Lust, G., and Smith, G.K.

A secondary effect of nutrition on hip dysplasia relates to weight gain. Simply stated, a diet excessive in calories causes excessive weight gain. The increased weight exerts additional mechanical stress on the growing joint, and for those dogs predisposed to dysplasia, the stress accelerates the disease.

Weight control is totally dependent upon owner compliance with dietary recommendations crucial to a successful outcome in the treatment of dogs with joint disease. Many older dogs with arthritis tend to be overweight as well. They are not able to exercise as they should because of joint pain. Therefore, they lead sedentary lifestyles, and sympathetic owners indulge their dogs with treats, thinking that the treats provide the dog with the only enjoyment in life.

Dogs on corticosteroid treatment for joint diseases develop increased appetites, and often gain weight when they can least afford to carry the additional burden. This vicious cycle starts with a joint disease that requires corticosteroid treatment, which increases appetite, which encourages weight gain, which stresses the joints, worsening the disease. Sometimes the treatment is worse than the original disease. Reasonable goals and diets can make weight control or loss easier on the pet and owner (it can be emotionally difficult to be the person responsible for a sedentary, injured dog's weight loss).

EFFECTS OF MUSCLE MASS

Dogs with significant pelvic mass have less incidence of developing hip dysplasia than dogs with little muscling. As should be expected, strong, well-balanced muscle support maintains congruity, not just of the hip joint, but all joints.

Physical or exercise therapy is known to combat joint stiffness, muscle atrophy, and bone resorption. Active exercise, such as swimming and walking, is more beneficial than passive manipulation or massage. But strict adherence to a veterinarian's treatment plan is important to success. Too much of a good thing can work against your goals. In order to be effective, physical therapy must be performed several times each day, gradually increasing the intensity and duration.

THE VITAMIN C HYPOTHESIS

Can vitamin C supplementation cure hip dysplasia? According to an article in *Outdoor Life* magazine (January, 1996), an English Pointer named Pinto was treated for hip dysplasia with vitamin C therapy. According to the article, B.J. Richardson, a Texas dog owner, relied on the work of California veterinarian Wendell Belfield of the University of California (Davis) to explore the use of vitamin C in combating the disease.

Dr. Belfield studied eight litters of German Shepherd Dogs, a breed known for high incidence of hip dysplasia. The study group included dogs that were affected by or were known carriers of hip dysplasia. Belfield fed high doses of vitamin C to the bitches throughout pregnancy and lactation. He found that none of the pups developed canine hip dysplasia during the study period.

Although not a truly scientific study, with controls and considera-tion of variables, the experiment may suggest a connection between vitamin C and the ability of the joint to remodel.

In the same article, a study by veterinarian L. Phillips Brown, of Cape Cod, Massachusetts, was cited. In a presentation to the National Conference on Holistic Veterinary Medicine, Dr. Brown discussed his findings from a double-blind crossover study of the effects of vitamin C on hip dysplasia. Brown concluded that "Seventy-eight percent of the dogs on 2,000 mg of Ester-C experienced improved mobility within four or five days . . . . About 60 percent of the improved dogs relapsed when Ester-C was discontinued . . . ."

The article discloses that x-rays of the dogs in the study showed evidence of loose joints or arthritis. According to the article, "Even Brown confirms that x-rays taken for his study reveal defective skeletal structures even after the Ester-C treatment."

Further investigation is needed into this subject, but as dog owners and veterinarians work together, observations may lead to discoveries.

BREEDING

Can we manipulate nature? Selective breeding of dogs has been prac-ticed for centuries, with the goals of producing dogs with desirable characteristics. We can produce a five-pound Yorkshire Terrier as easily as we can produce a stately Great Dane. Can we utilize our knowledge of genetics to produce dogs that are orthopedically sound? Screening of breeding stock and selective breeding are the keys in managing, if not eliminating, inherited orthopedic diseases in dogs.

According to the Orthopedic Foundation for Animals, canine hip dysplasia was first reported in 1935 by Dr. G. B. Schnelle, and the pop-ularity of working dogs, especially the German Shepherd Dog, raised public interest in the condition in the 1940s. As the field of radiology advanced in the '60s, so did the ability to diagnose structural maladies in dogs and other species, and cases of dysplasia were diagnosed more and more frequently.

Canine hip dysplasia is accepted as being an inherited disease caused by the interaction of multiple genes. According to OFA, "No environmental cause has been found, but environmental factors may influence the degree of expression of the genes within an individual." Therefore, reducing the frequency of CHD is dependent upon selective breeding of dogs with normal hips.

Twenty years ago, very few dog owners could pronounce dyspla-sia, let alone pose questions to their veterinarians about cause,

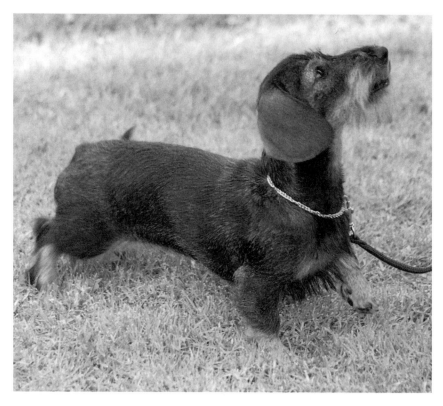

Selective breeding of physically and mentally sound dogs helps produce puppies more likely to avoid genetic diseases.

prevention, and treatments of the disease. Thanks to educational efforts within the veterinary community, today's informed pet owner understands the disease process and accepts responsibility for ensuring that their dogs avoid needless pain and suffering.

Breeders have been actively striving to eliminate the condition through genetic screening and selective breeding. And although progress has been seen in some breeds, others struggle to overcome alarming occurrence rates, particularly in large and giant breeds. What causes the condition? Some experts feel that popularity and increased demand for puppies in given breeds encourage opportunistic and/or unknowledgeable people to indiscriminately breed animals that are not thoroughly screened. However, even in pedigrees displaying multiple generations radiographically screened breeding stock, puppies continue to display hip dysplasia in alarming rates.

PennHIP® AND BREEDING

—Elizabeth LaFond, DVM
Post-doctoral research fellow in the laboratory of Dr. Gail Smith

When managing genetic diseases such as hip dysplasia, the objective of the conscientious breeder is to maximize the pairing of "good genes" by breeding dogs not overtly affected with or susceptible to the disease. Unfortunately, it is not possible to directly "see" the quality of a dog's genes from its physical appearance. Rather, the breeder relies on diagnostic testing (screening) to get a better picture of the genes (see illustration). This "picture" of the genes that a diagnostic test provides is known as the phenotype. In the case of hip dysplasia, the two most common phenotypes used to evaluate hip status are derived from different radiographic views of the dog's hips.

The hip-extended phenotype consists of an x-ray of a dog's hips taken with the dog lying on its back and its legs stretched straight out (as if it were a person lying down). In the case of OFA evaluation, the resultant x-ray is then subjectively evaluated by a panel of veterinary radiologists to establish hip status.

The PennHIP phenotype measures joint laxity from hip radiographs of a dog with all its muscles relaxed and the hips in the same neutral position the dog uses when standing normally. The x-ray is made with the femoral heads pushed out of the acetabula as far as they will easily go. A Distraction Index (DI) that is independent of dog breed, size and shape can then be calculated from the x-ray. The DI is an objective measure that corresponds to the percent of potential movement of the head within the acetabulum and is a number that will generally be between 0 and 1. DI of 0 would indicate a perfectly congruent joint and is what we see on the x-ray if we push the femoral heads deep into the acetabula, while a DI of 1 corresponds to the ability of the femoral heads to easily come completely out of the acetabula. So far, after radiographing more than 14,000 dogs from more than 100 breeds, even the healthiest hips have at least a small amount of detectable laxity (DI > 0). For the same dog radiographed in both the hip-extended view and the distraction view, there is *always* more laxity seen in the distraction view. As part of a complete PennHIP evaluation, the standard hip-extended view is also included to provide information about the presence or absence of arthritis.

Many traits we observe as being affected by environmental factors also have an underlying genetic component. For example, a dog's weight is partly influenced by environmental factors such as how much it is fed and how much exercise it gets. It is also influenced by genes:

Objectives of Selective Breeding

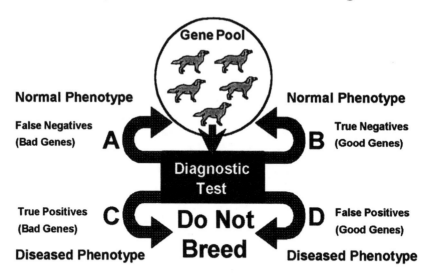

The role of a diagnostic test in improving the gene pool: The objective of any genetic diagnostic test is to use what can be seen (test results) to estimate what can not be seen (genes). Dogs enter the gene pool based on normal results of the test (arrow A or B). A perfect test would be capable of accurately separating "good genes" from "bad genes" on the basis of the phenotype (i.e., the test result), thereby quickly ridding the gene pool of bad genes (arrow B—good genes enter the gene pool; arrow C—bad genes are not reused). Unfortunately, no diagnostic test is 100% accurate. For example, a test result may wrongly exclude a dog that has a diseased phenotype from breeding even though it harbors good genes (arrow D). This would be an unfortunate missed opportunity, as some good genes would not enter the gene pool, however, this mistake would not appreciably harm the gene pool. Of greatest potential damage to the gene pool is a test result indicating that a dog has a normal phenotype even though it harbors bad genes (arrow A). Such a mistake would recycle bad genes through the gene pool, resulting in a steady-state level of disease in the offspring derived from that gene pool, despite the best efforts at selection. The frequency of disease coming from the gene pool will depend on the sensitivity of the test to detect bad genes. This sensitivity is directly related to the heritability of the phenotype used for screening, therefore, the higher the heritability, the better.

heavier parents tend to have heavier offspring. Heritability is a term geneticists use to describe the degree to which a trait (phenotype) is passed on from parents to offspring under the control of genes. In terms of using the phenotype as a diagnostic test or in a screening program, the more closely the phenotype represents the true status of the genes, the higher the heritability will be. Therefore, the higher the heritability, the more useful the trait (test) can be in guiding selective breeding.

Geneticists use various statistical methods to estimate heritability. Estimates are made by observing a large number of parents and their offspring and assessing how much resemblance there is between them. The more the offspring look like their parents (with respect to the phenotype under consideration), the higher the heritability will be.

Based on the studies out of the University of Pennsylvania, the PennHIP technology has promise to play an important role in breeding programs to combat canine hip dysplasia. Passive hip laxity, as measured by DI, has been shown to correlate very well with the later development of arthritis ("tighter hips are better hips"). DI has also proved to be a highly heritable phenotype in breeds of dogs in which heritability has been studied thus far. Therefore, given that "tighter hips are better hips" and tighter parents tend to throw tighter puppies, it makes good sense to breed tight-hipped bitches to tight-hipped dogs in order to decrease the number of dogs at high risk for suffering from the discomfort of arthritis.

How much improvement in hip status can a breeder expect when using DI as a selection criterion? The answer to this question depends, in part, on how much selection pressure the breeder can apply. Consider the relationship

$$\Delta \text{Generation} = h^2 \times (\text{Parent}_{ave} - \text{Population}_{ave}),$$

where

$\Delta Generation$ is the expected average change in litter DI after one generation,

h^2 is the heritability of DI,

$Parent_{ave}$ is the average DI of the selected parents, and

$Population_{ave}$ is the average DI in the entire population of dogs.

In English, this equation says that the amount of genetic change expected with each mating (ΔGeneration) is a product of the two factors on the right-hand side of the equation—selection pressure and heritability. Selection pressure will be bigger the more difference there is between the average DI of the parents and that of the population ($\text{Parent}_{ave} - \text{Population}_{ave}$). Heritability ($h^2$) is the measure of how much DI is affected by genetic rather than non-genetic factors. As can be appreciated from the relationship above, the higher the heritability of the phenotype, the more rapidly genetic change will occur. Breeders cannot influence heritability, but they can control how much selection pressure to apply (how different the selected parents are from the average in the population). Therefore, to the extent that breeders select breeding candidates, they can control how much improvement can be made in each generation.

For the most rapid genetic change, the breeder can decide to mate only the tightest-hipped dogs within the breed (those with the lowest DI) and then continue to inbreed for tight hips. This approach would maximize the difference between the parents and the population average (i.e., the selection pressure—the second term on the right side of the equation—would be big). There would therefore be a greater change in each generation given the same heritability. This approach raises concerns, however, that founding a breeding program on only a few dogs, and inbreeding on these dogs, would reduce the overall genetic diversity in the gene pool and might lead to a loss of some desirable traits while introducing some undesirable traits.

To avoid some of the problems associated with extreme selection, a moderate approach may be more appropriate, particularly in breeds that have few dogs with extreme hip tightness. In such breeds it may make more sense to choose breeding stock from the tightest half of the breed, thereby maintaining an acceptable level of genetic diversity while still applying meaningful selection pressure. The PennHIP evaluation report ranks each dog relative to other members of the breed, making it easy for the breeder to identify dogs suitable for moderate selection pressure. Eventually, the average of the population will become tighter and tighter and consequently, fewer and fewer dogs will be at high risk for developing arthritis.

In summary, the heritability of the phenotype measured using the PennHIP method has been shown to be high (approximately 0.50) for breeds thus far evaluated. Such information holds great promise for breeders who, by applying selection pressure based on the PennHIP phenotype, want to make rapid genetic change toward reducing the frequency and severity of arthritis in future generations of dogs.

CHAPTER 14

CONSERVATIVE
TREATMENTS

Whether physical therapy is an attempt to prevent the need for surgery, or a follow-up to surgical treatment, the treatment options offer tremendous benefits to diseased or injured dogs. Conservative treatment may be as simple as following the veterinarian's advice for limiting exercise (usually with confinement in a crate) or as complex as prescribed electronic stimulation and massage therapies.

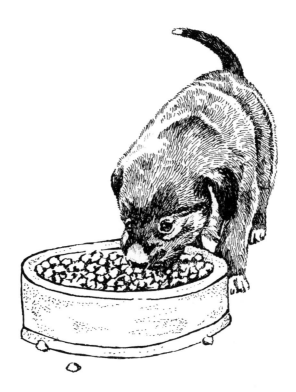

High volumes of calories, calcium, and protein are thought to contribute to the expression of genetic orthopedic diseases in large dogs. Avoid feeding puppies foods that contribute to rapid growth, and follow your veterinarian's recommendations carefully. *Illustration by Chris Hoy*

Diet and exercise can contribute to the development of orthopedic diseases, and dogs with known problems can benefit from specific diets and activities. However, conservative treatments are rarely the treatment of choice, so don't fool yourself into thinking that dietary changes will repair serious structural problems.

Why do some pets recover from injury, illness, or surgery more quickly than others? Why do some patients return to full function after surgery, while others with similar injuries and therapy experience limited success? Surgical aftercare can be as influential as surgery itself. When orthopedic surgery is completed, the skeletal structure has been dealt with; however, the *musculoskeletal* structure, which has also received a variety of stresses, must receive adequate attention for premium results.

Physical therapy is vital to treating pain associated with orthopedic problems and procedures. People treated for orthopedic problems would never be expected to return to normal activities without undergoing a program of physical therapy. Whether in the hospital or at home, therapies designed to improve flexibility, strength, and stamina should be prescribed by the doctor and implemented by trained medical staff. Principles for muscle repair are similar for people and dogs, so therapy should reflect those similarities.

Prior to the initiation of a physical therapy program, an orthopedic assessment should be done, including a complete examination of normal and abnormal limbs. The dog's normal limb can be a reference

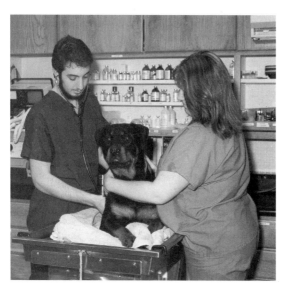

Dogs on restricted diets, prescribed exercise programs, or under doctor's care for any reason, should be closely monitored for general health, not just examined for the presenting problems. Stress can affect many systems and organs. *Photo by Leslie Bird*

point for comparison of short-term traumatic injury. However, the extra stress of body support and weight transfer, aggravated by long-term conditions, can cause changes in the normal limb.

The veterinarian should take each joint through its normal range of flexion, extension, and rotation, moving gently and smoothly. Pain or discomfort can be exhibited in varying degrees, from a mild tensing to a flinch or yelp.

Limb circumference and weight bearing status should be evaluated preoperatively, postoperatively, and throughout the duration of physiotherapy. Record and compare measurements throughout the treatment regimen. Use of a metric tape measure with specific landmarks on the body allows for measurement of muscle circumference, while maintaining consistency of measurements.

Weight bearing status can be subjectively evaluated through observation, with information recorded for comparison. Remember to include any observations regarding your dog's attitude, muscle strength, pain, gait, and ability to walk. Dogs with hind limb problems tend to be able to walk unassisted sooner than those recovering from forelimb trauma. This may be in part due to the increased proportion of body weight (60%) that is supported by the front legs.

PROCEDURES

Your veterinarian can choose from a variety of physical therapeutic procedures available to design a program to fit your dog's needs. Physical therapy should begin while your pet is hospitalized, and should extend into your home-care instructions. Your veterinarian will choose from therapies designed to address a dog's needs.

COLD THERAPY

After an injury or orthopedic surgery, cryotherapy (cold therapy) can be administered to relieve pain. This therapy is most effective when administered within seven days of surgery or injury. The cold temperature reduces the metabolic rate and temperature of the tissues, inhibiting the sensation of pain before the nerves can transmit it. Cold therapy provides a simple and effective first step in post-orthopedic surgery, physical therapy, often providing decreased muscle spasms and edema.

A simple, leak-proof bag filled with ice can be the basis of a therapy program; however, other choices exist. Continuous surface cooling blankets with circulating ice water or a liquid coolant are adaptable to companion animal use. Reusable cold packs wrapped in a damp towel may be applied for periods of 5 to 20 minutes or on an alternative schedule with 45-minute intervals.

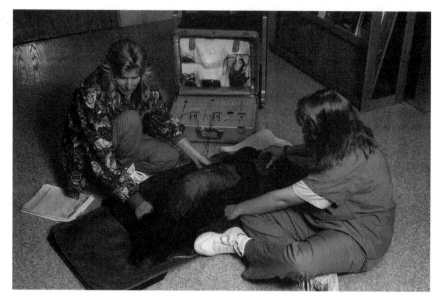

In-hospital physical therapy can involve sophisticated treatments, specifically pre-scribed to address a pet's most urgent needs. *Photo by Leslie Bird*

HEAT THERAPY

Conductive heat from moist hot packs or warm whirlpools provides effective pain relief and reduced muscle spasm. Benefits of heat application include mild analgesia, increased metabolic rate of the tissue, increased viscosity of collagen fibers, and relaxation of muscle spasms. Heat alone provides value, but often, the application of heat precedes massage or exercise, enhancing their benefits.

Pet owners can provide heat therapies at home, but radiant heat produced by long-wave rays (such as heating pads or hot water bottles) have limited tissue penetration. Short-wave rays (such as infrared lamps or generators) are more effective influences on lymph flow, nerve endings, and subcutaneous tissue; however, they must be used with caution to prevent the possibility of burn.Heating pads can also burn and should be wrapped in a towel.

Hot packs should be wrapped in a protective layer of warm, moist towels with application periods lasting 15 to 20 minutes. Monitoring skin temperature every few minutes reduces the chance of overheating the skin and inflicting accidental burns. Heating pads can also burn and should be wrapped in a towel.

Conversive heat (deep hyperthermia) is applied through the use of ultrasound waves. Mechanical vibrations are applied with a coupling medium using a contact (direct) or cushion (indirect) technique.

Ultrasound hastens healing while preventing fibrosis and muscle spasm. However, this therapy can cause dangerous burns to sensitive areas and is not recommended for eyes, spinal cord, brain, growing bone, heart, or reproductive organs.

Some cautions must be taken with heat-therapy protocols. Heat can be applied therapeutically 72 hours post-operatively, but immediate complications of vascular dilation and tissue swelling can occur if heat is applied too soon after surgery. Pets with heart disease, impaired circulation, or sensory nerve impairment require extra attention to prevent burns.

PASSIVE MOTION

Gentle mobilization of the joints has been found to be critical to the health of articular cartilage and to reducing the amount of muscle contraction and/or adhesions. Cartilage nutrition is an additional benefit from passive motion. Decreased muscle strength has been found in cases of injury and immobilization. Fibroblasts (the cells within connective tissue/muscles), which are affected by surgery, can be reoriented normal through muscle movement.

This reorientation decreases scarring and helps restore normal joint function. Passive motion should be initiated as soon as postoperatively possible, with the day of surgery, or the first day after, considered to be ideal commencement of the procedure.

During therapy sessions, the patient should be comfortable and relaxed, with the limb well supported. Passive range of motion should be performed slowly, with each joint of the affected limb cycled

Athletic dogs, like this Whippet, are prone to muscle injuries and should respond beautifully to physical therapy treatments.

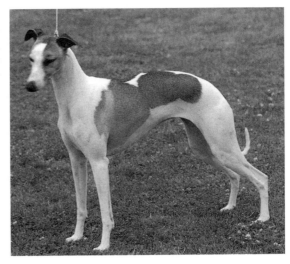

through its normal range of motion or until joint immobility limits movement. Passive range of motion should be performed only on sta-bilized limbs and joints (with internal or external fracture sites stabi-lized in a fixed position). Passive motion should be executed with 10 to 20 repetitions of movement completed two to three times daily. This form of therapy should be continued by the owner for two to three weeks after surgery.

DIGITAL MASSAGE

Physical therapies, such as digital massage, enhance circulation while loosening and stretching tendons. Pets find massage physically sooth-ing, often also relieving anxieties associated with hospitalization. There is little risk associated with digital massage, but health conditions that prohibit digital massage include infection, malignancy, or acute inflam-mation of the site being considered for massage. The size and condi-tion of the affected area, as well as the dog's response and progress, should be considered with regard to direction and pressure of the mas-sage stroke, the duration and frequency of treatment, and the rate and rhythm of the stroke.

There are three basic massage techniques and combinations that are used during treatment. The duration of massage sessions lasts between 10 and 20 minutes and should be performed every 24 to 48 hours. Begin and end each session with gentle stroking, monotonous movement which accustoms the animal to the therapist's touch. It is of uniform pressure with a light, sedative purpose. Called *effleurage*, it can also be performed with a heavy stroke for the enhancement of lymph and venous drainage. The stroke direction should be from the far end of the limb (or area) to the center or near end of the body.

Petrissage, a stronger form of massage, can be used on muscles as a group or individually. This technique incorporates a kneading or compression of the muscle from side to side, while moving the hand in the direction of venous return (that is, in the direction of blood flow, back to the heart). Benefits of petrissage include enhancement of cir-culation while stretching muscles and tendons to reduce adhesions and contracted muscles.

Friction, the third form of massage, aids in the absorption of localized fluid discharge, and the loosening of scar tissue or superficial adhesions. The skin is moved in small circular rhythmic motions while pressure is applied. Friction encourages collagen to realign in the proper direction.

Exercise can be a helpful form of controlled physical therapy. It coordinates muscle groups performing like and opposite actions, aid-ing in strengthening and maintaining functional use. This action improves balance, stability and coordination in the dog. With the benefits of exercise, complete paralysis can gradually progress to slight paralysis, weak ambulation, and finally to normal movement.

The forms of exercise range from passive- to active-assisted, and end with active-resistive. When passive exercise is indicated for paralyzed or weakened patients, a body sling or cart can provide support while improving sensory awareness and muscle strength. This form of passive-assisted exercise can also include helping to support the patient's weight through the use of a harness or the buoyancy of water.

Assisted exercise re-educates muscles and aids in neurologic recovery. *Encouragement and praise is an important aspect of assisted exercise,* benefiting disabled pets psychologically. Wheelbarrowing and repetitive limb placement aid in the concentration of weight bearing stress to improve neuromuscular function.

Active resistance strengthens muscles and increases stamina and coordination. Joints should be moved through their range of motion, with the

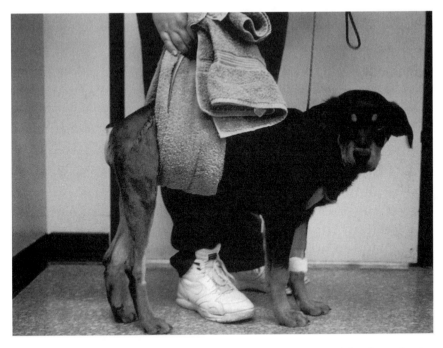

Use of a sling, shown here as a towel, enables the therapist to aid the dog in beginning exercise. The therapist can assist the patient with mobility, while the dog challenges the muscles to resume working.   *Photo by Leslie Bird*

therapist applying gentle resistance. A gentle, non-painful, yet annoying stimulus applied to the digits (e.g., slight toe pinching) will cause the animal to withdraw the limb. Repetition of this action, with resistance applied first to the farthest part of the body (distally), and then closest to the body (proximally), will strengthen limb muscles. Downward pressure placed on the pelvis causes an active resistance and increases information from the nerves regarding body position. Cooperation from the dog can be obtained by praise and positive reinforcement.

Balance can be a form of active resistance by gently pushing at the hip or shoulder, forcing a redistribution of weight. Release of pressure causes the pet to return to the immediately previous balance and weight distribution. This balancing action should be repeated several times from each side.

Numerous short exercise sessions are better than one long session and induce better cooperation from the dog. Be sensitive to your pet's responses while pushing them to their performance limit without exceeding the boundaries of good sense. Begin with a five-minute period of exercise and work up to 30 minutes if approved by your veterinarian.

Leash walking in short circles or figure-eight patterns improves muscle strength. Offering diversified surfaces, such as grass, carpet, or sand varies muscular workload and coordination. Patients who resist bearing weight on a disabled limb can be encouraged to use it by making use of the functional limb uncomfortable. (This can be done by taping a marble or plastic bottle cap under the toes for the exercise period.)

Repetition of sit and stay commands strengthens hind limb muscles, particularly the stifle. This strengthening results from a stretch-and-hold repetition of the associated musculature. Pets recovering from front-limb surgery can benefit from a slow walk on a gentle incline or stairs. These inclines encourage better leg flexion and extension. Wheelbarrowing, or lifting the patient onto the affected front or rear limbs, is another form of exercise encouraging weight bearing.

Swimming offers non-weight bearing exercise with vigorous range-of-motion opportunities. The buoyancy and hydrostatic pressure provide upright support, enabling the pet to stand or walk in water, often sooner than gravity would normally allow. Offered in a controlled and closely supervised environment, warm water (102 to 105 degrees F) provides conductive heat as well as kinetic heat, which is transformed to thermal energy (heat within the muscles).

Whirlpool therapy is beneficial for the treatment of decubital ulcers as well as stiff joints and adhesions. During the treatment period, whirlpool therapy can provide a combination of physical therapy methods. Passive and active-assisted therapies, and different types of massage as described above, can be performed while the patient is experiencing superficial hyperthermia. The water is kept at 102 to 105 degrees F, and should be level with the pet's chest. Dogs can be provided with assisted walking in the whirlpool, and can also experience some active resistance while moving against the water flow.

Caution must be taken, however. It is important to disinfect the whirlpool tank between uses to reduce the spread of bacteria. When using either whirlpool or swim therapy, encourage the pet to urinate and defecate prior to the exercise session. Whirlpool treatments should be withheld until 5 to 20 days after surgery to allow healing of incisions. Pets receiving whirlpool therapy sessions should be constantly monitored, with the flow of water directed *away* from the affected area.

OTHER THERAPIES

Exercise restriction is a simple and effective method of reducing orthopedic pain. Post-operatively, pets should be kept in a confined area, away from other animals. Reducing voluntary activity allows for the natural process of healing to occur, while preventing further damage to the musculoskeletal system (which can result from the animal trying to compensate for a disability).

Limiting the dog to an area with just enough space to lay down or turn around is vital for successful healing of orthopedic procedures (such as total hip replacement or pelvic reconstruction). When combined with controlled leash walks and physical therapy, exercise restriction allows for optimal healing conditions for orthopedic patients.

PATIENT RESPONSE

A substantial part of convalescence takes place in the home, and home care is vital for the success of a physical therapy program. Therefore, it is important for owners to learn to properly perform the prescribed therapies. Owners must avoid the temptation to pity their pets, and should offer support and hope instead. Owners may lack elaborate equipment, but the stimulation of massage, and the effects of hot/cold packs and exercise, will dramatically effect recuperation.

Response of the dog to physical therapy treatment should be a continuation of the initial patient assessment. Measurements of the limbs can indicate a mild response or a lack of any response to therapy. It is important to maintain consistency in this objective evaluation process. The owner should keep a daily record of the pet's response to treatment on a calendar or in a log book.

Although these are subjective observations, the information can be valuable if kept in two-week reference frames, rather than as a comparison of day-to-day progress. In this way, slow progress can be bet-

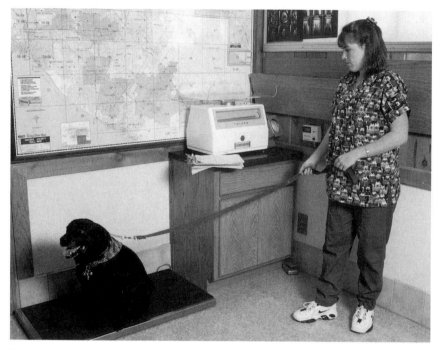

Exercise programs contribute to many aspects of a patient's health. Weight control, improved coronary function, and enhanced temperament can result from regular exercise.   *Photo by Leslie Bird*

ter appreciated over a period of time, offering encouragement to you as both the owner and daily care provider.

At each veterinary re-check appointment, therapy should be re-evaluated. Your veterinarian should schedule postoperative examinations at 5 to 7 days and again at 10 to 14 days to determine patient progress and to alter therapy when indicated. Owners should resist temptation to self-prescribe therapy, because damage can occur when inappropriate therapies are selected.

CHAPTER 15

PAIN AND ANALGESIC THERAPY

"Is my dog in pain?" Pet owners ask this question every day. We know that animals experience pain, but unlike humans, they cannot tell us where the pain is located, what it feels like, its strength, or how long it has been occurring. To better understand animal pain, we need to recognize the signs, how it functions, and review appropriate treatments. We must also recognize the "why" of pain.

Like some humans, animals can be stoic and not let pain bother them until it becomes so severe that they cannot avoid showing it.

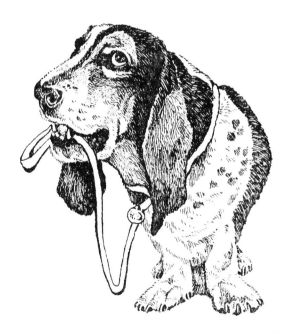

Dogs cannot verbally relay information about pain and suffering. Monitoring a dog's reactions to daily activities can tell a lot about the dog's comfort level. Reluctance to go out on daily walks may signify underlying joint, muscle, or spinal damage. *Illustration by Chris Hoy*

Others enjoy sympathy. A dog may limp all day until allowed out to chase rabbits, suddenly running and jumping without the slightest appearance of discomfort. Is this dog in pain even when running? Yes. However, the excitement of chasing rabbits can release the dog's endorphins, which temporarily dull the pain, much like a good analgesic.

An *analgesic* is a drug or therapeutic method that brings pain relief, or decreases the ability to feel the sensation of pain (the awareness or perception of a stimulus that is potentially damaging to tissue). Pain is associated with subjective feeling of discomfort or unpleasantness. An animal will try to relieve pain by favoring the affected area (exhibited by lameness). Limitation in activity or movement of a painful limb provides time for tissue healing and reduces the possibility of further damage. Therefore, pain is important by being the incentive to limit movement of an injured limb.

Animals cannot easily communicate their discomfort to us; therefore, we often neglect to treat their pain. A change in a dog's behavior may provide the only indication of pain, and keen observation skills aid in identifying pain. Although the perception of pain is similar between individuals, pain tolerance fluctuates greatly even within the same patient. The perception of pain varies, based on:

- States of anticipation

- Focus on the situation

- Stress level

- Counter-irritation

- The pet's emotional state

There are three categories of pain: *acute* (sharp or severe), *chronic* (long-term), and *generalized.* Acute pain is associated with signs of vocalization, rapid heart rate, panting, salivation, dilated pupils, and chewing of the painful area. Chronic pain may result in weight loss, lethargy, groaning, whimpering, sleeplessness, loss of appetite, or aggression. Animals may pace or exhibit restless behavior in an attempt to find a pain-free position. Generalized pain may be acute or chronic and is usually associated with restlessness and irritability.

ANALGESIC THERAPY

The goal of analgesic therapy is *not* always to eliminate *all* pain; sometimes it is only to reduce it to a tolerable level. Certain levels of pain serve a useful purpose and may not be treated. For example, discomfort limits activity and promotes healing in patients with intervertebral disc disease.

Excessive pain and most postoperative pain warrants treatment. For postoperative pain management, the analgesic should be administered *before* seeing clinical signs of pain. Just as in human medicine, preventing the pain is more effective than trying to relieve agonizing pain later.

Increasing the dose or combining analgesics (unless prescribed) not only fails to enhance the effect, but may be dangerous and cause serious health problems, including bleeding ulcers, kidney or liver failure, and clotting disorders.

Analgesics act on peripheral pain and are used for the treatment of mild to moderate pain, such as that accompanying degenerative joint disease. However, mild analgesics are of no benefit in the treatment of acute or visceral (abdominal) pain. Categorized among these pain relievers are local anesthetics, nonsteroidal anti-inflammatory drugs *(NSAIDs)* and glucocorticoids.

Local anesthetics include topical sprays or creams, injections of an analgesic, or nerve blocks (such as epidurals). Local analgesics are not frequently used for numerous reasons, such as not being as effective,

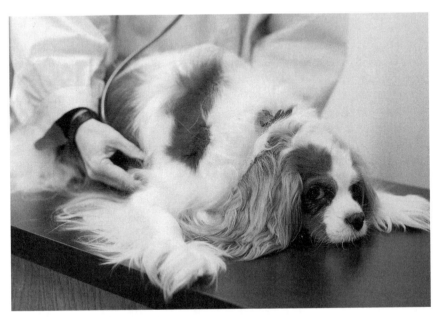

Avoid the temptation to "self medicate" your dog. Every dog for whom pain relief drugs are prescribed should undergo a basic physical examination. This practice is especially critical when dealing with infirm or geriatric patients. *Photo by Leslie Bird*

having a shorter duration, or allowing the dog to use a limb. These could cause further damage to the locally anesthetized area (injections in a joint). Nerve blocks, such as epidurals, should only be used in conjunction with sedatives, because of a dog's inability to understand the reasons that certain areas of the body are numb. This can be very confusing and upsetting to a dog.

NSAIDs have been used by veterinarians for many years for treatment of inflammation and pain. The drugs often provide good response; however, occasionally an unfortunate toxic effect occurs. Because NSAIDs are available over the counter, owners sometimes use them indiscriminately and at higher-than-proper doses. The variability in the response to medications is often misunderstood by owners, who simply believe that the medication that has relieved their own aches and pains will similarly relieve their pet's discomfort.

Before giving any drug—even those available over the counter—owners should consult with their veterinarian to determine appropriateness and dosage. Most dog owners are often unaware of drug absorption rates, distribution of the medication within the body, paths of excretion from the body, individual variations, or interactions that may occur with currently prescribed medications and/or preexisting diseases.

Discuss the type of inflammation/pain (acute, chronic, or generalized) seen in your dog with your veterinarian, and consider the body system that is causing the symptoms of pain (soft tissue, musculoskeletal).

Many dogs experiencing pain from arthritis or other orthopedic problems are geriatric (senior citizens). Internal organs, such as the kidneys, liver, and heart should be evaluated with a geriatric blood screen prior to using NSAIDs. Because the body clears drugs through these organs, the geriatric blood screen is critical in identifying preexisting conditions that might influence the practical use of NSAIDs. Furthermore, gastrointestinal effects can occur with the use of NSAIDs. Pets exhibiting digestive problems, or having recent histories of stomach upset or diarrhea, should avoid NSAIDs.

Many NSAIDs exhibit anti-prostaglandin action. The prostaglandins produced in synovial joints are a part of the inflammatory response and cause pain. The acid pH of inflamed tissues draws NSAIDs to affected tissues, and the antiprostaglandin action reduces tissue sensitivity to pain.

NSAIDs are inappropriate for use in some dogs. Antiprostaglandin NSAIDs are contraindicated when the dog is in a prostaglandin-dependent state, including conditions such as congestive heart failure, liver failure, dehydration, diarrhea, general anesthesia, diabetes mellitus, von Willebrand's disease, urinary obstruction, or any renal disease. NSAIDs can affect the platelets in the blood, which cause coagulation and clotting of blood. Prolonged use of nonsteroidal anti-inflammatory drugs may cause bone marrow suppression, electrolyte and acid base imbalances, convulsions, coma, or death. *A rule with NSAIDs is to use as little as necessary to relieve pain.* This lessens any potential side effects.

DRUG OVERVIEW (NSAIDs)

Acetaminophen: This is a coal-tar derivative for analgesic and fever-reducing benefits. There is no prostaglandin inhibition in this NSAID. Use in cats is contraindicated due to the toxic or fatal effects in that species.

Adequan (Polysulfated Glycosaminoglycan): A cartilage-protecting agent in dogs. Adequan can inhibit the function and release of several enzymes in the joint spaces, giving damaged cartilage time to repair itself. The best time to begin therapy is soon after trauma occurs, before biomechanical degeneration begins. There have been no toxic effects reported in dogs; however, Adequan is not currently licensed by the FDA for use in dogs in the United States.

Aspirin: Historically, aspirin has been used in dogs for the management of degenerative joint disease. The use of buffered (maalox-coated) or enteric-coated aspirin, "ascriptin," may reduce some of the incidences of stomach upset. *Do not use aspirin to treat cats. It can be toxic and fatal.*

DMSO (Dimethyl Sulfoxide): Approved for topical use in dogs, DMSO causes local vasodilation and analgesia. It is used in cases of bursitis, arthritis, and musculoskeletal injuries. It is considered relatively nontoxic when it is used topically, although clinical signs of halitosis (bad breath), vomiting, and changes in the eye may appear if toxic levels are approached.

Cosequin: The building blocks to synthesize synovial fluid and cartilage matrix are contained in this neutraceutical. Capsules may be sprinkled on moist food or given orally; however, noticeable response or reduction of clinical signs may take up to one month to be observed. Although this is not considered a drug, it contains agents that protect the articular cartilage without the side effects of the NSAIDs or steroid medication commonly used to manage joint diseases.

Ibuprofen: Although this drug may be used in dogs for treatment of inflammation associated with musculoskeletal disorders, caution is recommended. *The drug's elimination time from the dog's body is very slow, and toxic levels can be reached rapidly. Other NSAIDs are preferable.*

Naproxen (Naprosyn-Syntax): Naprosyn is not approved for use in animals; however, it has been used in dogs. There have been reported cases of severe gastric ulceration, perforation, and hemor-rhage associated with its use. Elimination time in dogs is very slow. Use with caution if at all for pain associated with arthritis, degenerative joint disease, and inflammation.

Feldene can be a very effective analgesic, but severe gastric ulcer-ation and renal disease have been associated with high doses. Other NSAIDs are preferable.

Arquel (Meclofenamic Acid) is a useful analgesic for chronic osteoarthritis. It is best given with a meal to try to prevent gastroin-testinal bleeding.

Phenylbutazone has been found to be less effective as an anti-inflammatory drug than some of the other NSAIDs, but tends to have good analgesic effects for postoperative pain. There is a high incidence of toxicity with this drug, especially when the animal's liver metabolism is accelerated by phenobarbital, griseofulvin, and phenytoin.

Banamine (Flunixin Meglumine) frequently is administered for postoperative pain relief, for treatment of toxic shock, and as an anti-inflammatory. In horses, it can be an effective analgesic for stomach pain (it is the only NSAID analgesic used for visceral pain). *It is not rec-ommended for use in cats.*

The use of all drugs should be cautiously judicious. Physical man-ifestation of stress (gastrointestinal upset/bleeding/ulcers) may aggra-vate the toxic effects of NSAIDs. Most dogs in need of analgesia are under stress.

GLUCOCORTICOIDS

Glucocorticoids are anti-inflammatory steroids. They reduce inflamma-tion and other factors that contribute to pain, but *they do not have direct analgesic effects* and cannot be substituted for analgesics in pain control. In some situations they satisfactorily alleviate pain.

Steroid anti-inflammatory drugs alleviate pain, but may accelerate the degenerative processes in degenerative joint disease. Their use should be restricted to severe cases. There are numerous NSAIDs that are well tolerated and can provide significant relief.

Steroids can be very useful when secondary inflammation (and thus pain) is not a part of the disease, yet needs to be controlled. Intervertebral disc disease is one in which steroids can be very helpful. They can reduce the cord compression and associated pain by decreas-ing inflammation.

The steroid dosage, frequency, and duration must be followed cor-rectly, because too much or too frequent steroid use can be harmful to the intestinal tract and liver. Stopping the medication abruptly can cause an entire body crisis in that the body needs time to adjust to making its own steroid again. Therefore, a gradual tapering off of the steroid is necessary.

When used judiciously (as with all medicine), steroids can be very beneficial to the treatment of many orthopedic problems. Avoid concurrent use of NSAIDs with other NSAIDs or with glucocorticoids. Toxic effects are greatly multiplied when used in conjunction and can be life-threatening.

SPINAL CORD ANALGESICS

Analgesics that act at the spinal cord include anesthetics such as opiates or xylazine, which your veterinarian would administer in a controlled situation. Opiates are most effective for treatment of pain in internal organs, rather than for a sharp acute pain.

Glucocorticoids are used frequently for spinal disease to alleviate pain, and to reduce inflammation that is usually the cause of the pain and damage to the cord.

ACUPUNCTURE

Acupuncture is one of the oldest methods of pain relief known, and has been used in the treatment of animals as well. In some studies acupuncture stimulates the nerve tissue and local tissue cells, releasing endorphins or neurohormones. Some endorphins relieve pain, while others give the animal a sense of well-being. The body's natural cortisones are released, and increased circulation to the joints or areas receiving treatment may occur in response to acupuncture. All of these help to alleviate pain.

ELECTROSTIMULATION

This procedure stimulates the function of nerves through the layers of skin at acupuncture sites. It enhances the electrical activity of damaged tissue while increasing the rate of healing. The electro-acuscope restores the normal electrical activity of damaged nerve axons by stimulating regrowth. Treatments are cumulative, and correct the signals transmitted by the nerves without blocking them.

NEUROMUSCULAR STIMULATION

Electronic neuromuscular stimulation has been used for several years in treating small animal patients. Its benefits include pain control of both acute and chronic neurologic conditions. When limbs have been stabilized with casts or bandages, the stimulation pads can be placed over selected muscle groups to activate muscular contraction during periods of generalized immobilization. Neuromuscular stimulation is aimed at diminishing muscle atrophy, while providing increased blood circulation, muscle tone, and range of motion. The increase in blood circulation aids in reducing fluid accumulation and inflammation at surgery sites.

RADIATION THERAPY

Radiation therapy is usually used for dogs with osteosarcoma tumors that have advanced beyond the stage considered most responsive to chemotherapeutic or surgical success. Often, metastatic tumors are inoperable because of multiple tumor sites. Cancer patients experiencing pain or dysfunction associated with bone tumors can find relief through palliative (pain-relieving) radiotherapy. It is used most often for treatment of metastatic bone tumors (those that develop in multiple sites beyond the primary tumor).

Fractions (portions) of radiation can be administered to the tumor at intervals based on the individual patient's needs. Pain relief often begins after the first fraction of the prescribed radiation. Palliative therapy does not provide tumor control, but offers pain management for pets with painful, localized disease. The duration of pain relief extends up to several months for some individuals.

CHAPTER 16

SURGICAL REPAIR PROCEDURES

A diagnosis of orthopedic disease or injury often results in a recommendation of surgery. Certainly no one is pleased to hear of their pet's need for surgical procedures, but the good news is most orthopedic conditions can be corrected with surgical intervention. Diagnosis of an orthopedic disorder does not have to mean that a pet endures a lifetime of suffering or imminent loss of life. Advances in veterinary medicine allow pets to benefit from new technologies. Nowhere is this more evident than in the diagnosis and treatment of orthopedic disease.

As with any complex medical procedure, you should seek the most qualified help available to perform these highly specialized procedures. Although primary care veterinarians can perform many surgeries with

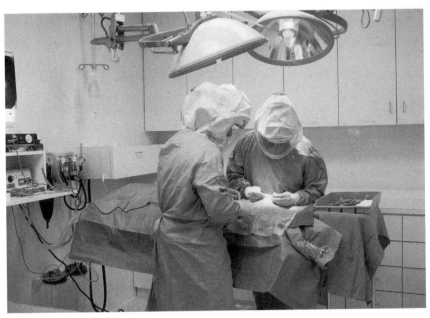

The decision to undergo surgery should never be made lightly, but most orthopedic surgeries are quite safe when performed by a skilled surgeon.

considerable skill, many orthopedic procedures require special skills and specialized equipment to attain optimum results.

Opinions sometimes vary regarding the "best" treatment option for a given condition or a given dog. Often variables such as the general health and activity level of the dog or an owner's financial ability to pursue treatment affect the decision-making process. Furthermore, the recommended treatment may reflect an individual school of thought, and different professionals may offer varied opinions about treatment. Therefore, the pet owner should attempt to thoroughly understand his or her dog's disease, treatment, and prognosis. A second opinion may disclose valuable insights and relevant decision-making facts. Trust your judgment; if you are unsure of the best course of action for your dog, seek answers within the expansive veterinary community.

Depending upon the complexity of a required surgery and the interest of your primary care veterinarian, you may choose to have your dog's regular doctor perform a simple orthopedic surgery. Or, you may select a specialist who has pursued extensive formal training in the field of orthopedic surgeries, understudying leaders in the field, reading journals, and attending continuing education seminars. Veterinarians differ in their skill level and interest in surgery, so choose a surgeon based on the complexity of the procedure at hand. Some fracture repairs and ligament reconstructions may be performed by your regular veterinarian. Complex procedures, such as spinal surgeries and joint replacements, require the experience and training of highly skilled surgeons.

Board certification from the American College of Veterinary Surgeons (ACVS) is given to those who meet the stringent standards of admission. ACVS requires applicants to complete post-doctoral training and a residency at an accredited institution. Residents in these programs attend formal classes and work in clinical situations that give them hands-on experience with specialized surgeries. ACVS applicants must prove their specialized competency and perform satisfactorily on practical and written examinations.

PROCEDURES

What happens during surgery? Understanding the procedures a dog will undergo may help owners understand the progress of disease, treatment, and recovery. Veterinarians should explain the recommended procedure to your satisfaction during your presurgical consultation.

OSTEOCHONDRITIS DISSECANS (OCD)

OCD can be treated medically or surgically, depending upon the severity of the disease. How does a veterinarian determine the treatment

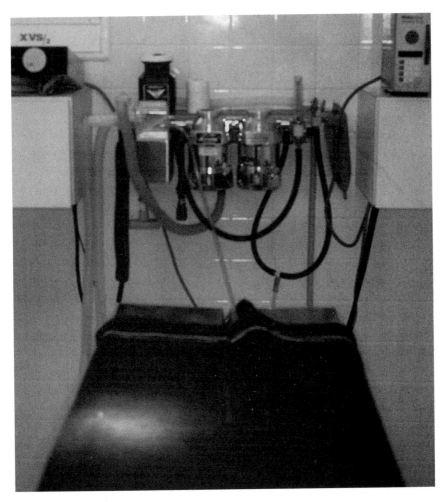

Modern veterinary surgical suites are equipped with anesthesia and monitoring equipment to maximize safety.

route? Guidelines have been established to define or categorize the criteria for choosing treatment. An OCD lesion can be managed medically when the following conditions are present:

- The lesion in the joint measures less than 1 to 2 mm wide and 1 mm deep.

- The lesion has no flap.

- The dog lives pain free.

Otherwise, the lesions must be surgically repaired or else they will not heal, and secondary osteoarthritis will ensue. This standard can be applied to OCD treatment of any joint.

Medically treated cases should be closely monitored, with attention paid to any changes in the size of the lesion. Although medical treatment may first be attempted for treating OCD, surgical repair may become necessary if the lesion enlarges beyond the size guidelines established above.

Surgery has two goals: to remove loose fragments or flaps and to curette the defect in the articular cartilage.

During surgery, the joint is exposed and the articular flap and/or joint fragment is removed by flushing the cavity. The edges of the articular cartilage defect are rounded to alleviate stress areas, and the defect itself is curetted (scraped) down to bleeding bone. The curettage speeds up the normally slow healing process of cartilage by actively engaging the subchondral bone. Before closure, the joint must be flushed thoroughly with a sterile solution to remove all debris and blood.

Postoperatively, one week of absolute exercise restriction should be followed by three weeks of gradual, slow leash walks. The animal should then be back to (or close to) full function and normal activity, but prognosis varies with the site of the lesions. Most dogs with humeral head lesions are able to function well within one month of surgery. OCD lesions at other sites are not as predictable, but surgery still remains the preferred treatment for clinically evident lesions.

UNUNITED ANCONEAL PROCESS (UAP)

All cases of UAP should be treated surgically, but controversy exists regarding the ideal age at which surgery should be performed. If possible, wait until the dog is no longer in the fast-growing phase (four to eight months). In some cases, however, surgery should be scheduled as soon as possible, regardless of the dog's age. These cases include patients with severe pain, non-weight bearing lameness, or those exhibiting secondary degenerative changes.

Surgical management entails removal of the ununited anconeal process or reattachment of the process to the ulna using a compression screw. Which surgery is preferable? The answer may vary. Some surgeons feel the elbow becomes more stable by reattachment of the process, others feel removal of the process has no detrimental effect and may lessen complications. In cases that include osteoarthritis, surgery must include removal of osteophytes. Flushing the joint is the final step in the surgery. Postoperatively, a bandage may be placed on the surgery site for three to five days. Exercise must be restricted for the first two weeks. Over the next two weeks, slow, gradual leash walks may be initiated.

An uncomplicated UAP that receives proper surgical repair prior to osteoarthritis has an excellent prognosis. With osteoarthritis present, surgical repair still carries a good prognosis, but these patients may limp slightly or intermittently.

FRAGMENTED CORONOID PROCESS

A fragmented coronoid process in the elbow must be surgically removed to prevent secondary osteoarthritis. Surgical management involves removal of the fragment and curettage performed on the surface where the fragment originated. As usual, the joint should be flushed with a sterile solution to remove blood and debris.

The approach to the elbow joint involves (medial) incision with joint exposure gained by muscle separation, or in extreme cases osteotomy of a collateral ligament of the joint.

Postoperatively a bandage may be placed on the surgical site for three to five days. Exercise restriction must be enforced for four to eight weeks, depending on the surgical approach.

Response to surgical removal of the fragmented coronoid varies with the degree of osteoarthritis present before surgery. However, even if osteoarthritis is already present, surgery should lessen further degenerative changes.

FRACTURE REPAIR

Fractures often occur as a result of accidents and trauma sustained from twists, blows, or crushing. Successful repair of broken bones often requires quick response in stabilizing the dog and transporting to a veterinary hospital.

Fractures are classified according to multiple factors:

- Stable (main fragment ends are in contact)
- Unstable (ends not in contact)
- Open (bone fragment extends through the skin, is contaminated, or open to the outside)
- Closed (intact skin over the fracture site)

Fractures can be *single* or *multiple*. Types of fractures include:

- Greenstick
- Fissure

- Transverse

- Oblique

- Spiral

- Comminuted

- Impacted (compressed)

- Avulsion

- Physeal (growth plate)

- Condylar

- Or a combination of the above

While all fractures require immediate attention, not all fractures are solely trauma-induced, and many conditions affect the prognosis for recovery. The presence of preexisting disease can cause fractures and influence the type of repair chosen. Such disease may be systemic, such as hyperparathyroidism preventing normal calcium deposit in the bone thus causing weak, brittle bone fractures, often seen in the jaw bone and mouth. A diabetic will experience problems with wound/soft tissue healing, which directly affects bone healing. A dog with cancer can develop pathological bone fractures in relation to a tumor in the bone.

Disease may be concomitant with orthopedic disease, such as that seen in a young puppy hit by a car, damaging its hip joint. The impact causes the hip to luxate, and if the puppy suffers from hip dysplasia (even if the disease was never clinically evident), just replacing the hip in the dysplastic joint will not accomplish the goal of returning the joint to "normal." The joint most likely luxated because of the preexisting dysplasia.

Injuries to more than one limb can severely complicate recovery. Older dogs are at risk when a fractured limb occurs in conjunction with severe arthritis of the opposite limb. If both limbs are "out of order," such a dog won't have a limb to stand on, unless the fracture repair is very stable. A large dog with multiple limb fractures may temporarily lose the capacity to walk, which could become a very serious complication, depending on the dog and the owner.

The breed and age of the patient also play a role in the prognosis and choice of repair techniques. Toy breeds are more difficult to treat, as circulatory complications and nonunion occur more frequently in Toy breeds than in others. Also of special concern is the immature animal with the possibility of growth plate damage sustained during the trauma, which could cause growth deformities.

When dealing with a fracture, one must also consider that the fractured bone does not exist alone in its environment. The surrounding soft tissue and vasculature play major roles in bone healing. A bone will not heal, regardless of surgical excellence, if surrounding soft tissue does not also heal. Surgical repair of the bone is sometimes delayed to allow the traumatized soft tissue time to begin its healing process.

The function of the limb or joint can be compromised by the degree of soft tissue trauma, hemorrhage, and subsequent scar reaction with resulting ligament, tendon, or muscle damage or adhesions—even when the bone has healed beautifully.

Surgeons should discuss complication risks with their clients to avoid conflicts after surgery. Many owners would consider the surgical repair to be a failure if a complication prevented full recovery for their dog. Dog owners should inquire about risks and possible outcomes of surgery, along with the surgeon's opinion about the likelihood of concurrent conditions affecting a potential surgical procedure.

An orthopedic surgeon has many options available for repairing fractures. He or she can choose from many techniques and implants, including intramedullary pins, external fixators, wire, bone screws, bone plates and screws, casts, and splints.

The implant or techniques may be used as a primary repair tool or in combination with other options, when secondary supports are deemed necessary. Although casts and splints are usually not used with internal fixation devices, they can be effective for stabilizing metatarsal or metacarpal fractures.

The method of fixation chosen depends on the type, location, and complicating factors (infection, missing tissue, previous failed repair, systemic disease) of the fracture. The method of fixation is not nearly as important as the philosophy behind its use.

The first decision in regard to fracture repair involves whether to use an *open technique* or a *closed technique.* The fixation method of choice will depend on the type of fracture, and proper application of the appropriate technique improves the chances for a positive surgical outcome.

An open technique entails a surgical opening to the fracture site. Open techniques for fracture repair achieve better fracture reduction, but can add to soft tissue damage risks. Stabilization methods most commonly utilized include intramedullary pins (can also be used for closed reduction), bone screws, bone wires, and bone plates with screws.

A closed technique (or external coaptation) is a reduction of the fracture without penetrating the skin. The fracture is manipulated via traction, rotation, or by bending to a stabilized, aligned reduction. The fragments are then held in place by an external fixation method, such as casts, splints, bandages, slings, or a Kirschner-Ehmer apparatus.

External coaptation can only neutralize the angular and rotational forces applied to the fracture or joint being immobilized. Compression and tension forces will continue to affect the site. If compression or tension are of primary concern, then external coaptation is not the treatment of choice.

There are five major types of external coaptation available:

- Casts

- Splints

- Padded bandages

- Slings

- The Kirschner-Ehmer apparatus

Casts are tubular structures that are molded to the animal's limb. Indications for casts include closed, simple transverse fractures of the radius, ulna, or tibia; closed, highly comminuted fractures of the radius, ulna, or tibia; unstable dislocation of the carpus, tarsus, and elbow; and as an adjunct postoperatively to ligamentous injuries.

Several products are available for use as cast materials. Plaster of paris has been used for many years, but it creates a heavy cast that degenerates quickly when immersed in water. Newer products (hexcelite, Vetcast) are lightweight, strong, porous, and waterproof. However, special equipment is needed for application or removal of these types of external coaptation devices.

Splints are usually molded to one aspect of the limb with bandaging covering the remainder of the circumference. *Spoon splints* or *half casts* are indicated for fractures of the metacarpus, metatarsus, or digits; fractures and dislocation of the carpus; and greenstick fractures of the distal radius or ulna. *Lateral splints* can be made of yucca board, thin plywood or cast material that is cut to the shape of the limb. These are best used on greenstick fractures of the radius, ulna, and tibia; as an adjunct to internal fixation of the radius, ulna, and tibia; and as transition coaptation from a full cast to complete weight bearing. A *modified spica splint* is made of cast materials and is used as an adjunct to internal fixation of the humerus and femur and in minimally displaced fractures of the humerus and femur in young animals.

A *Robert Jones bandage,* a heavily padded cotton supportive dressing, is used for early immobilization of massive soft tissue wounds, early immobilization of fractures below the elbow or stifle, and for reduction of severe soft tissue swelling. It is most commonly used prior to, or immediately following surgery.

Slings prevent weight bearing on the front or rear limbs. The *Velpeau sling* is used in the thoracic limb following reduction of a shoulder luxation; in scapula fractures; and as an adjunct to internal fixation of elbow or humeral fractures. The *Ehmer sling* is used on the pelvic limb and will maintain abduction and internal rotation of the femur and prevent weight bearing on the limb. It is used following reduction of luxated hips; to maintain reduction of supra-condylar fractures in young animals; and for luxation fractures of the tarsus.

There are disadvantages of external fixation. The reduction of a fracture is less precise. Exercise and use of the limb muscles are limited, and disuse atrophy is likely. Care of the cast or splint may be difficult.

A *Kirschner-Ehmer apparatus* provides stability of bone fragments without placing implants in the fracture site or immobilizing adjacent joints. Therefore, this is useful for treatment of open, comminuted, or infected fractures. It is also a useful technique used to avoid further soft tissue damage. A Kirschner-Ehmer apparatus, an external skeletal fixation device, utilizes pins placed through the skin into or through the bone to the opposite side of the bone, perpendicular to the limb. Pins on either side of the fracture line are then externally connected by one or two vertical bars to form a rigid frame.

Aftercare of all external coaptation devices is extremely important. The veterinarian must educate the client on the at-home care of splints and casts, and he or she should confirm the effectiveness of instruction with regular examinations of the animal. The pet owner should check daily to see that the coaptation device remains dry, clean, and does not wear excessively.

Areas of the skin that become irritated from contact with the cast or splint should be treated with the appropriate medication. The feet or toes should be gently palpated for signs of edema or pain. Any foul odors or changes in position of the splint or cast should be immediately reported to the veterinarian. Unexplained fever, depression, or inappetence are also reasons for an immediate examination.

Most internal implants should be removed when the fracture has healed. Some exceptions exist, including lengthy removal procedures, potential causes of infection, potential soft tissue trauma, and when anesthesia presents excessive risk to the patient.

Small implants need not be removed, and implants in dogs with systemic illness should remain if they are not causing problems. Pelvic plates should be left intact, as well as plates in dogs more than 10 years of age. If an implant in any case loosens or becomes infected, it should be removed. Obviously, external fixators are always removed.

Returning to activities should be carefully executed. Excessive exercise leads to fixation failure. Not enough exercise leads to healing failure. It is important to follow instructions provided by the surgeon for rehabilitating the recovering dog. Postoperative care includes exercise restriction with slow leash walks only for four to eight weeks. Re-examinations by the surgeon are very important, usually occurring at one week, two weeks, four weeks, and eight weeks postop. These examinations give the surgeon the opportunity to correct any problems (such as fracture complications, implant loosening, or fracture displacement—all of which most commonly occur when postoperative instructions are not followed) before they can cause permanent damage.

SURGICAL REPAIR OF TENDONS

Surgery for a ruptured tendon usually involves end to end anastomosis (the joining together of the two ends). Sometimes tendon lengthening or tendon grafts are necessary.

Surgical repair involves or consists of three goals:

- To minimize adhesion formation
- To provide a strong union
- To maintain tendon length

Most tendon injuries in dogs are caused by trauma, involve open wounds, and are compound in nature. Therefore, to minimize inflammation, the tissue must be handled with care and cleaned thoroughly. If the wound is infected, the tendon should be labeled and repaired after the infection is controlled. Otherwise, immediate surgical repair is recommended.

Following surgical repair, a device that braces the repaired site from the outside of the body (external fixation) is sometimes applied to ensure stabilization. Postoperative care involves strict confinement with no exercise. The length of time varies with the degree and site of the lesion.

Prognosis also is variable, but the companion dog can usually be returned to function, whereas the "professional" canine athlete may be compromised.

SURGICAL REPAIR OF LIGAMENTS

Damage to ligaments ranges from slight sprains to tears. Determining the extent of damage will clarify the appropriate treatment.

Ligament sprains without tears may be treated with immobilization with or without external coaptation and strict confinement for 4 to 6 weeks. Normal activity should not occur before 10 to 12 weeks.

Surgical repair of a torn ligament involves suturing end-to-end (anastomosis) to restore the natural arrangement. When ligaments suffer extensive damage or display severe weakness, the ligament may require anchoring to its bone of origin or insertion. Screws and wires, or sutures in a figure-eight pattern around the screw anchor the ligament to the bone.

Because the tensile strength of ligaments varies with age, dogs respond differently to similar traumas. An adult dog is more likely to tear the ligament under similar circumstances. An immature dog may suffer an avulsion (a portion of bone to which the ligament attaches breaks off in response to the tension on the ligament rather than the ligament itself tearing). Avulsions should be reattached with a screw or tension band wire.

Postoperatively, it is important to keep the affected joint immobile. This is usually accomplished with external devices, such as splints or external fixators, for five to six weeks. After removal of the external device, activity should be restricted for another six to eight weeks while allowing weight bearing. Weight bearing promotes stronger healed tissue, provides nutrition to the cartilage, and restores pliability of the periarticular tissues. Prognosis varies, but function can eventually be fully restored, even in the athletic dog.

SURGICAL REPAIR OF MUSCLES

Trauma causes muscle injury, varying from bruising to disruption. Conservative treatment involves aggressive physiotherapies and rest; however, advanced muscle tears require surgery. Bruising and swelling may interfere with the surgical procedures, therefore it is usually recommended to rest the dog for two to three days prior to surgery to allow inflammation and hemorrhage to subside.

Surgery involves removal of hematomas and devitalized muscle, and anastomosis of the muscle. Depending on the severity of the damage, the surgical procedure could be simple and quick or complicated and time-consuming.

Short, slow leash walks may begin seven to ten days postoperatively with a gradual return to running over three to four weeks. Athletic training should not resume for three to four months. Prognosis for return to athletic function can be good.

PATELLA LUXATION

Luxation of the dog's patella (kneecap) can occur medially or laterally. The surgical treatment procedures selected to correct patella luxation vary with the individual case and the grade of luxation, but there are certain procedures common to all. Due to the infrequent nature of lateral patella luxations, discussion of patella luxation repair will focus on medial patella luxation (MPL).

The goal in performing knee surgeries is to recreate or stabilize the components of the knee so that the joint can complete a normal or near normal range of motion and support the weight of the patient. Common goals for most MPL surgeries are reinforcement of the patella in the trochlear groove (the groove in the femur in which the patella rides) and realignment of the quadriceps muscle.

Securing the patella in its functional position prevents it from popping in and out of the joint, which causes pain and reduces functionability. Reinforcement of the patella is accomplished by tightening the lateral aspect of the joint (medial displacement of the patella tears or stretches the lateral joint capsule) with local connective tissue or suture materials. Once the patella glides in place appropriately, the surgeon will assess the condition of the joint capsule and excessive capsule tissue from repetitive stretching in a dysfunctional joint will be excised.

In a normal knee, the patella rests in the trochlear groove. If the trochlear groove is shallow or the medial ridge of the groove is worn down from repetitive luxations, reconstruction of the groove may be necessary to allow the knee to function properly. However, need is usually not determined until the condition of the groove can be visualized and evaluated during surgery.

When the surgeon determines that the trochlear groove is damaged or too shallow, repair efforts begin. The procedure involves lifting the articular cartilage from the joint, slowly scraping the subchondral bone until an appropriate groove is made, and replacing the cartilage. Most dogs undergo the procedure without complication; however, older dogs with brittle cartilage may require special attention.

A dog with brittle cartilage should undergo the wedge technique, in which a wedge is cut from the groove and carefully removed. A second wedge is cut into the underlying bone to create the necessary groove, and then the first wedge with the articular cartilage is replaced. The wedges enable the bones to seed together and function as a unit.

As some animals develop, a malaligned quadriceps muscle pulls the patella, forcing it to luxate, and a normal groove fails to develop. When quadriceps malalignment causes MPLs, surgical realignment of the quadriceps muscle is indicated, which involves transplanting the tibial tuberosity (insertion at the quadriceps or patella tendon), thus shifting the patella to the center of the groove. The transplanted bone is held in place by a screw and wire, stabilizing the joint and allowing it to function properly.

The majority of cases involving dogs with luxating patellas are correctable with just the patellar reinforcement and quadriceps realignment; however, complications evolve. In some cases, patellar luxation can be directly linked to other conformation defects. For example, stress placed on the knee may originate from a need to relieve a damaged hip joint from carrying burdensome weight. If a dog continually throws unusual weight to the knee, the knee joint will be adversely affected. Correction of specific conformational defects that have led to or contributed to the MPL (such as hip dysplasia) may be necessary to prevent the joint from further damage. The surgeon should discuss the plan for correction of each underlying problem and determine the order of procedures based on the individual dog's condition.

Dogs usually recover very quickly from knee surgeries, and some dogs attempt to use the joint on the very day of surgery. Most are walking within 48 hours after the procedure. Postoperative immobilization is not necessary unless both stifles undergo surgical correction simultaneously. In the case of simultaneous, bilateral repair, a soft padded bandage is placed on each limb for five days.

Exceptions to the rules do occur, and the surgeon should advise the dog owner of these situations. For example, dogs who undergo tibial tuberosity transplantation may require four to eight weeks to start walking on the affected limb, and owners should remain patient during their rehabilitation.

Exercise restriction in a confined area should be enforced for three to four weeks, at which time a progressive increase in activity begins and leads to normal activity over the following four weeks. Full return to function should commence by eight weeks, although the dog will continue to improve postoperatively for eight to sixteen weeks, depending on the severity of the MPL.

Surgical repair of medial patella luxations generally leads to a successful outcome. If corrected early, the prognosis is excellent.

RUPTURED ANTERIOR CRUCIATE LIGAMENT (RACL)

The knee joint should always be surgically stabilized after complete rupture of the anterior cruciate ligament. The medial meniscus also may be torn acutely at the time of injury to the cruciate ligament, but more often it is damaged as a result of chronic instability. The damaged meniscus may make a recognizable clicking noise while the dog walks. The damaged meniscus is removed when the cruciate ligament is repaired. Surgical repair of the ligament and meniscus will usually result in a reduction of lameness and a decrease in the degenerative changes in the joint, thus delaying or preventing the onset of arthritis.

Many approved surgical techniques are available, with a common goal of joint stabilization and prevention of the abnormal movement that causes degenerative changes and ultimately arthritis. Surgical repair of the joint usually quite successfully allows the dog to return to normal activities; however, in the large-breed dogs, a surgically repaired knee may never be as strong as it was before injury.

The numerous surgical repair techniques may be classified as penetrating the joint capsule (intracapsular) or stabilization without penetrating the capsule (extracapsular). The goal of all techniques is to reproduce the normal biomechanic function of the ligament.

Intracapsular repair involves replacement of the cruciate with material (synthetic or autogenous) as close to its normal location as possible. Prior to placement of this material, the remnants of the damaged cruciate ligament and meniscus, as well as any osteophytes, are removed to prevent degenerative changes in the joint and to accommodate regeneration of a fibrocartilagenous meniscus that will replace the original. Proper regeneration cannot occur if the meniscal remnants are left in. Unfortunately, the developed (regenerated) meniscus is not as strong as the original.

Frequently, the graft dies or the synthetic material breaks, but this usually occurs after the material has been replaced by collagen and formed into a ligamentous structure. (If a synthetic radiodense material is used, the material is commonly reported to be incidentally seen on x-rays and found to be broken. Once again, this is an incidental finding on x-rays taken for other problems, not because the stifle is a problem.) Initial stability is provided by the material, whereas long-term biologic replacement is provided in the formed ligament.

Extracapsular repair techniques are used more frequently in small dogs and involve stabilizing the joint with sutures outside the joint capsule in order to eliminate cranial and rotational instability. Extracapsular techniques are quick and provide excellent stability, although they result in some abnormal joint movement and thus degenerative changes may occur over time. Even if external stabilization will be performed, some feel the joint should still be opened to evaluate the intraarticular structures and to remove damaged tissue.

Large, heavily muscled dogs should almost always undergo intracapsular repair. If both knees contain a ruptured cruciate, one side is repaired with an intracapsular technique and the second side is stabilized with an extracapsular suture until the first side heals. Eventually, the second side undergoes intracapsular repair when the first knee has healed enough to support the dog's weight.

Frequently, an injury will result in a partial cruciate tear. These injuries should be repaired as a complete tear, because the ligament is no longer functional.

Postoperatively, the limb is *not* bandaged. Exercise is restricted to crate or small room confinement for the first four weeks with a slight increase in activity between four and eight weeks; unrestricted activity is usually allowed after eight weeks. Undue stress on the stabilization material during the first four to six weeks after repair may lead to stretching of the material and joint instability. Therefore, not only is it important that the surgery be done correctly, but also that the postoperative instructions are strictly followed.

SPINAL LESIONS

Spinal lesions can occur anywhere along the spinal cord and even within the cord (neoplasia, hemorrhage, or inflammation). Lesions will most commonly be the result of trauma, intervertebral disk disease (IVD), spontaneous embolus, neoplasia, or instability. (Spinal lesions are discussed here because they can cause or mimic orthopedic disease.)

The basis for the surgical repair does not completely lie within the cause of the lesion, but in the lesion itself, the location and duration of the lesion, and the number of lesions. The severity of the lesion is more pertinent to the prognosis than the actual type of surgery performed.

Cord tumors can occur in the cord itself, in the lining of the cord (dura), or in the outside of the dura. If the tumor lies within the cord, surgical resection is not recommended, radiation or chemotherapy would be the treatment of choice. If the tumor is in the dura or outside the dura, a surgery to excise the tumor will also decompress the cord. A laminectomy exposes the canal and the mass unless the mass lies within the dura, then a durotomy (opening cut into the dura) is also performed. When the entire mass cannot be removed, follow-up radiation or chemotherapy may be recommended, and prognosis can still be very good.

Trauma-induced spinal lesions (automobile accidents, falls, big dog/little dog fights . . .) usually consist of vertebral fractures or dislocations. Surgical repair is undertaken to stabilize the area and decompress cord compression when present. If the fracture is stable and spinal cord compression does not exist, conservative therapy under a watchful eye is warranted. Immediate surgery would be necessary if the status were to change.

Cervical fractures need surgical fixation much less frequently than elsewhere. Rest and a neck brace may be satisfactory treatments. Thoracolumbar fractures/luxations, however, almost always require surgical correction.

Surgical approach to the spinal column in the neck region can be ventral (front) or dorsal (back), but the majority of lesions (85%) will be most easily attainable via a ventral approach. All other areas of the spinal column are approached from the back.

Vertebral fracture repair employs the use of pins, wires, screws, and plates. Decompression is usually accomplished by realignment of vertebrae; therefore, a laminectomy (removal of the vertebral arches to visualize and decompress spinal cord lesions) is not routinely performed. This is important because of the removal of the dorsal arch (laminectomy tend to make the column more unstable.

Postoperatively, most surgeons prefer strict crate rest/confinement for four to eight weeks rather than body casts or braces, which tend to be uncomfortable and cause the dog to squirm or struggle. For the best course of rehabilitation, passive physical therapy should be initiated immediately, followed by swim therapy and slow walks when able.

Prognosis varies with the extent of existing spinal cord damage. While the bones can be put back and made to heal, the spinal cord might not. It is very important to know what to expect for future function before surgery.

Time, and occasionally anti-inflammatory drugs, are the therapeutic necessities for treating embolic disease. Embolic disease does not require surgical intervention unless there exists severe cord swelling, which may benefit from a durotomy. A *durotomy* removes the sheath surrounding the cord, which due to the cord swelling may be inadvertently causing compression.

Prognosis is usually good, but will vary with location of the embolus and severity of the post-embolus inflammatory response, hemorrhage, or necrosis. For recovery to occur, evidence of improvement usually will be seen within a week.

Good nursing care and passive physical therapy are necessary until the dog is able to walk. There are no exercise restrictions, except to not allow overactivity or the dog to hurt itself trying to do things it is not yet capable of doing. Otherwise, once the patient is able to do something, allow it, within reason.

Although therapeutic procedures for intervertebral disk disease (IVD) vary from rest with or without medication to surgery, the surgical methods have one goal—to remove disk material compressing he spinal cord (infrequently, the sole purpose of surgery is to do a fenestration—remove the degenerated nucleus pulposus before it compresses the cord).

Cord decompression begins with gaining access to the spinal canal. A procedure termed a laminectomy or hemilaminectomy accomplishes this. A laminectomy is performed by removing the bony arches of the vertebra. For a hemilaminectomy, only a portion of the arch is removed. This allows visualization of the compressed cord and allows the surgeon access to the extruded intervertebral disk material. The disk material is then removed and the surgery site closed. A laminectomy will leave the vertebrae more unstable than before surgery. Therefore, in certain situations, preexisting instability may eliminate this as an option. In a dog without spinal stability problems, this postop instability is not significant.

More than 75% of dogs under 50 pounds with IVD develop the disease between the 11th thoracic vertebra to the 2nd or 3rd lumbar vertebra. This occurs because the thoracolumbar (TL) region is the most unstable area of the spinal column. The thoracic region is the most stable, protected by the paraspinal muscles, the thoracic girdle, and the ribs. The lumbar region has only the paraspinal muscles for protection and is thus the most vulnerable region. This large difference in protection makes the TL junction very unstable, thus the most common place for disk disease. Due to this instability, surgeons will, if possible, do only a hemilaminectomy in this area, making it less unstable afterward.

Dogs larger than 50 pounds develop disk disease most commonly at the lumbosacral junction, due to its propensity for instability. In this area, only a dorsal laminectomy may be performed because of the location of the nerve roots.

A fenestration is frequently performed at the same time as a decompressive laminectomy and infrequently as a primary surgery. Fenestration involves making a hole in the disk annulus and removing degenerate nucleus material before it has the opportunity to rupture or protrude and compress the cord. The surgeon may fenestrate the intervertebral spaces around the laminectomy site.

Postoperative care will vary in the degree of nursing care necessary. Recumbent dogs will require soft, clean bedding periodically turned to prevent ulcers, bladder expression, and possibly feeding assistance. An ambulatory dog will not need such intensive care, but will require four weeks of crate or small room restriction and on-leash walks to urinate and defecate, followed by another four weeks of gradually progressive, slow leash walks. During this time, passive physical therapy, electrostimulation, acupuncture, massage, or swim therapy may all be helpful. Once ambulatory, active physical therapy takes over, but many dogs still benefit from a good massage!

The prognosis is dependent on the chronicity, severity, and location of the disk. The vast majority of dogs with disk protrusion or rupture will recover to at least a functional dog, if not a normal dog.

Just about all patients with clinical signs of a spinal cord lesion undergo myelograms (a contrast radiographic study of the spinal canal and cord—contrast is injected into the spinal canal to outline or delineate the cord and any lesions). A small risk of allergic reaction to the contrast material exists. For this reason and because magnetic resonance imaging (MRI) offers a more accurate and detailed analysis, MRI is the preferred diagnostic method. With the increased use of MRI, myelography use will change, but will still be used for dynamic testing.

Lumbosacral (LS) instability or congenital malformation may lead to stenosis and compression of the nerve roots (the cord ends prior to the LS segment). Surgical stabilization and decompression is the treatment of choice. Stabilization is achieved by fusion of the LS junction and decompression by dorsal laminectomy in conjunction with LS foramenotomy. (A foramenotomy consists of widening the foramen or funnel through which the nerve roots exit the canal.)

Crate confinement and strict exercise restriction for an average of four weeks is essential to obtain satisfactory results. The following four weeks consist of continued confinement with slow, gradual walks. Depending on the status of the patient, it must get good nursing care. The urinary bladder may need to be manually expressed three times daily if the dog is unable to urinate independently.

A good prognosis can be given in most cases.

ATLANTOAXIAL SUBLUXATION

The atlantoaxial (C_1C_2) joint allows little flexion. During subluxation, the amount of flexion exceeds the normal amount and results in dorsal displacement of the axis and spinal cord compression. Early intervention can maintain spinal cord function and allow recovery. Surgical correction involves decompression of the cord as well as stabilization of the joint.

The surgical approach is from the dorsal neck. Removal of bone from the atlas and axis allows decompression. Stabilization of the joint is most commonly achieved by placing wire through a natural arch in the atlas and through two holes drilled in the axis. This wire is tightened with the head in a natural position. The stabilization does not hinder normal head and neck movement.

Postoperatively, strict crate rest must be enforced the first week. This leads to four weeks of general rest—no running, jumping, or playing. Some passive physical therapy may be recommended during this time. For the first few days postop, some patients may require a neck brace.

If detected and treated early, the prognosis is excellent. Complications are minimal, and even a chronic case usually has a good outcome when stabilized.

CERVICAL VERTEBRAL INSTABILITY (WOBBLERS SYNDROME)

The primary problem in a dog with wobblers is cervical vertebral instability, but this leads to spinal cord compression through two methods. The first type of compression can be caused by hyperplasia of vertebral ligaments. The hyperplasia is the body's attempt to stabilize the areas.

The second way the cord suffers compression can be from disk protrusion. This chronic instability leads the disk to degenerate and eventually protrude or rupture.

Surgical treatment must address all three conditions when possible and necessary. Irreversible spinal cord injury can occur quickly; therefore, once a diagnosis is made, treatment (medical or surgical) must be initiated immediately. Treatment for each case varies with the individual, the chronicity of the disease, the presence of a damaged disk, the number of areas involved, and the degree of compromise.

The surgeon generally will approach from the ventral neck if there exists a ruptured disk and from either way (dorsal or ventral neck) if not. The latter would be dependent on location and preference.

There are numerous techniques described for stabilization of the cervical spine. These techniques include the use of screws, wires, pins, or a bone plate. Generally, stabilization may be achieved by placing a cortical bone graft between the unstable vertebrae and a bone plate or pins holding the graft in place.

A hemilaminectomy or dorsal laminectomy allows exposure and removal of damaged disks compressing the cord. A fenestration (prophylactic removal of disk material from possible problem areas) may be performed to prevent future disk complications. The laminectomy also allows decompression of the cord caused by ligament hyperplasia.

Postoperative immobilization in a cervical stabilization collar or splint will encourage fusion of the unstable vertebrae and allow the spinal cord time to heal. The patient should undergo enforced rest for eight to twelve weeks. Physical therapy consisting of passive-limb range of motion, slow walking with or without a sling, whirlpool baths, or swimming may be helpful. When the patient is ambulatory, slow walks with a harness (a neck collar should never be used again) will aid recovery. Running and jumping should be prohibited for twelve weeks.

The prognosis depends on several factors. The chronicity of the lesion is one factor. More chronic cases carry more significant potentials for irreversible cord damage and worse prognoses than other cases. In the functional dog, surgery is recommended to prevent further progression and more nerve function loss. The severity of the spinal cord compression is also a factor. If diagnosed and treated early, the prognosis for a functional dog is good. A performance dog will most likely not return to competitive function.

HIP DYSPLASIA

In deciding what to do with a dog presented for hip dysplasia, consideration should be given to several factors. Among these factors are the age and size of the dog, the clinical signs associated with the dysplasia, and the severity of the disease. The main reasons for performing surgery are:

- To relieve the pain
- To return the patient to normal or near normal function
- To prevent or reduce the progressive degenerative changes

The goal of surgical intervention would be to restore congruency and stability of the hip joint. This will halt or diminish osteoarthritis and allow the dysplastic dog to run, play, and function.

Numerous surgical procedures exist to treat hip dysplasia. These are pelvic osteotomy (unilateral or bilateral), femoral neck lengthening, intertrochanteric osteotomy, femoral head and neck resection, pectineus tendonectomy, and total hip replacement.

The hip is a ball and socket joint. The acetabulum is the socket half; it is a part of the pelvic bone. The ball half is the head of the femur—the long leg bone.

Pelvic Osteotomy

This surgical procedure changes the orientation of the acetabulum in relation to the femoral head. The surgery provides more dorsal coverage of the femoral head by the acetabulum. This solves the problem of insufficient dorsal acetabular rim coverage of the femur, which allowed luxation.

The surgery is done mostly in young dogs (four to thirteen months of age) where the primary problem is subluxation, and the femoral head and acetabulum have few secondary changes. The actual age of the dog is less important than the good condition of the joint surfaces.

This procedure can be done when the acetabulum is shallow. Since the young dog still has some ability to remodel, the acetabulum will deepen as weight bearing occurs.

There are a few contraindications for pelvic osteotomy. If osteoarthritis is already present, the pelvic osteotomy surgery will rotate the acetabulum but will not alleviate the pain induced by the already present arthritis, thus the surgery would not be clinically successful. Another case leading to a failed surgery would be if the rim loss is excessive. A surgeon can rotate the acetabular cup 30 to 35 degrees. After that, sufficient cartilage breakdown would lead to further degeneration and osteoarthritis.

The pelvic osteotomy is performed by cutting the pelvic bone in three locations, rotating the acetabulum, and placing a specialized bone plate to stabilize it while it heals.

Historically, the surgery is done on one side at a time. Recently, great results have been seen with repairing both hips at the same time. The benefits of simultaneous bilateral repair are great. The dog and owner undergo only one surgery, anesthesia, and set of postoperative restrictions. The dogs tolerate the postoperative pain equally for uni-lateral and bilateral and are ambulatory within hours postop. Most important, the second hip is not lost to arthritis (and thus a total hip replacement or salvage technique) while waiting for the first hip to heal (during which time the second hip would be the sole weight-bearing limb). (This obviously creates added stress to an already suboptimal joint.)

Postoperatively, strict crate confinement must be enforced for four weeks, then house confinement and exercise restriction (no running, jumping, playing, or stairs) for four more weeks. During the second four weeks, slow, gradually progressive leash walks begin. By eight weeks, no restrictions are placed, and by six months, normal function should exist.

Technically, once the pelvic bone heals, the bone implant (plate) can be removed. This is usually not done unless the implant causes a problem, such as screw migration or infection. Otherwise, the implant is left in and causes no problems for the dog, thus avoiding a second surgery for the dog. The most common cause of screw migration is owner failure to restrict activity during healing.

Prognosis for lifelong success with a pelvic osteotomy is excellent if the patient is suitable and the surgeon is competent with this surgery.

Femoral Neck Lengthening

This is a procedure that increases the femoral neck length and thus gives the femur a better angle of approach or lever in relation to the cup.

The femur is partially split along its long axis, and wedges are placed in the split. Pins and wires stabilize it. This surgery can be done only in young dogs without already present osteoarthrosis.

This procedure is not common. It is performed on dogs felt to have a shortened femoral neck. By improving the ball coverage, developing hip dysplasia and secondary osteoarthrosis may be halted.

Intertrochanteric Osteotomy

This surgery is primarily indicated for dogs between eight and twelve months of age who have subluxation of one or both hips without osteoarthrosis. The surgical objective is to reduce the angle of the femoral neck, to correct abnormal rotation of the femoral neck, and to increase the length of the femoral neck. With these changes, the femoral head is forced more deeply into the acetabulum, providing a more stable hip joint. If necessary bilaterally, the surgeries are usually separated by about six weeks.

A specially designed plate and screw are used to stabilize the femur after a wedge of bone is removed and the proximal fragment is rotated to correct the abnormalities. Postoperative care for intertrochanteric osteotomy.

Intertrochanteric osteotomy is a relatively new procedure; prognosis at this time appears to be good, but follow-up radiographs have shown progressive, subclinical osteoarthritis.

Femoral Head and Neck Resection

This surgical procedure has been used for quite a few years. It involves removing the head of the femur, thus eliminating the "ball" in the ball and socket hip joint. The purpose of this surgery is to relieve the pain associated with osteoarthritis in a degenerative hip joint. It is a salvage procedure. It is a less expensive but less reliable alternative to a restorative surgery.

The surgery is performed only if the patient is in pain, a restorative surgery is not possible or is cost prohibitive to the owner, and the patient weighs less than 20 kg (it can be done in heavier dogs, but not as successfully).

Following surgery, the dog should be pain free, but the range of motion of the hip joint will be decreased and the joint will be less stable. A fibrous scar joint forms between the femur and the cup. The abnormal ball and socket joint is sacrificed to eliminate pain and preserve or improve limb function. The surgical limb will be functionally shorter than the non-surgical limb, although most likely this will not be clinically evident.

Postoperatively, the patient should use the limb as soon as possible. Passive physical therapy or swimming are used to maintain as much flexibility as possible. The fibrous joint formed greatly limits flexibility. The patient must not be allowed to become overweight. It is not recommended to do both hips simultaneously; the second hip should be postponed until the patient bears weight on the first hip.

This surgery can be very successful in small dogs and in cats. Smaller breeds will have less gait change than larger breeds.

Pectineus Tendonectomy

The pectineus muscle extends from the pelvic bone to the femur on the inner ventral aspect. Its purpose is to adduct the limb. A pectineus tendonectomy includes removing a portion of the tendon that attaches the pectineus muscle to the femur. If the tendon is only cut, it tends to form a fibrous reattachment and thus becomes functional again.

This procedure is not a cure for hip dysplasia, it is done to allevi- ate pain. Pain relief results from allowing increased abduction of the limb (which allows better articulation) and relieving tension on the joint capsule. This surgery does not stabilize the joint, thus osteoarthro- sis generally continues and pain usually recurs with time.

Exercise restriction is enforced for two weeks after surgery. This procedure is useful for dogs whose owners cannot afford reconstruc- tive or replacement procedures and for dogs with degenerative changes from advanced hip dysplasia.

Total Hip Replacement (THR)

This procedure has been in clinical use for more than 13 years. It is in- dicated for any dog over 10 to 11 months of age, once the trochanteric growth plates have closed, who is limping or having pain related to osteoarthrosis of the hip joint. The head of the femur is excised, and a hole is made down the center of the femoral shaft (this is where the stem of the ball portion of the implant is placed). A prosthetic cup is positioned on the acetabulum. Once these are complete and cemented in place, the ball is placed in the cup.

Manufacturers have created prostheses in five stem sizes, allowing prosthesis implantation in dogs as small as 14 kg (30 pounds) and as large as the giant breeds. Four sizes of acetabular cups are available, and a detachable ball and stem is more recently available. The new device offers not only variable stem sizes, but also variable ball depths (diameter remains standard) to allow for various femoral neck lengths. The ball and stem are made of cobalt-chrome; whereas the cup is high density polyethylene plastic.

Postoperatively, the patients are confined in crates and limited in activity for four weeks following surgery (no running, jumping, play- ing, or stairs). No activity more strenuous than a walk is allowed. Then gradual return to full function is allowed.

Total hip replacement should not be done in dogs without hip- induced lameness or pain and in dogs with systemic infection present, neurologic disease of the hind legs, or concurrent orthopedic problems.

The success rate is about 95% plus for this surgery, which means the dogs are pain and limp free and dramatically improved over the preoperative state. This procedure can be performed bilaterally with eight to ten weeks wait between surgeries. However, 80% of dogs will only need to have one hip replaced even if dysplasia and osteoarthrosis exist in both hips, because the total hip replacement provides enough relief that surgery on the other side becomes unnecessary.

Many working and pet dogs have been returned to full activity following total hip replacement. The prosthesis provides the dog with a normal ball and socket joint, allowing the femur to maintain its normal position (thus the hind leg is able to generate maximum propulsion forces during locomotion). The prosthesis offers a lifetime of pain free, normal activity for most patients.

Other options include two procedures that are being evaluated for treatment of hip dysplasia. These are BOP shelf arthroplasty and cementless total hip replacement, which are discussed in the final chapter.

SALVAGE PROCEDURES

A salvage procedure can best be described as a surgery that allows function, but does not preserve normal anatomy. The amount of function allowed varies, but will be limited. Most salvage procedures are performed when a previous procedure has failed, when an owner cannot afford the restorative procedure, to alleviate pain, or if the salvage procedure leaves the pet just as functional as the restorative, yet the restorative is not available or more costly. (An example of the latter would be a dog weighing less than 25 pounds needing a total hip replacement. However, implants are not available for that small of a dog, therefore a femoral head ostectomy is performed. This will leave the dog just as functional as the THR would have.)

The goal of most salvage procedures is to allow a dog and owner an option other than euthanasia or a life of pain. The salvage procedure is never the ideal. Restoring a joint or limb is always preferable, but may not always be possible. Surgeons try to maximize restoration and minimize salvage, but salvage procedures need not be considered the consequence of failure. Salvage techniques can give many pets and pet owners a second chance at a pain free existence. The lifestyle may need to change some to accommodate for the limited function, but this seems a small price to pay for most people who want to keep their families intact and their family members free of pain.

There are three common categories of salvage surgeries: arthrodesis, amputation, and excision arthroplasty.

Arthrodesis is the surgical fusion of a joint. Arthrodesis would be indicated for crippling arthritis, irreparable trauma to a joint, especially if there is a loss of tissue (i.e. shearing wounds, common when a dog is dragged by a car), malignant neoplasia, or irreparable instability. Arthrodesis of a joint will usually leave the pet with an obviously "choppy" gait, but more importantly free from pain.

The carpal and shoulder joints are very amenable to fusion. The gait may be only slightly "choppier" than normal, and success of the surgery is usually more likely than if a restorative process is attempted. Restorative surgeries of the carpus and shoulder frequently fail. Vertebral arthrodesis can also be done without limiting function. All other joints, if arthrodesed, will not result in the near normal level of function like shoulder or carpal arthrodesis, but will lead to a functional, happy dog.

Amputation, or surgical removal of a limb or tail (or a part thereof), is indicated when the limb hinders more than helps the dog. An unacceptable level of hindrance would be caused by a limb in which the dysfunction is beyond repair, in which exists a malignancy with metastatic potential (as yet not having occurred), or in which there is severe pain unresponsive to treatment, interfering with the dog's quality of life.

Amputation of a forelimb is usually accomplished at the scapula level, removing it with the rest of the limb. It is a fairly nontraumatic surgery in that the scapula thoracic joint is only muscle.

Amputation of a hind limb can be done one of two ways. For a cancer lesion, the surgeon disarticulates the limb at the hip joint, removing the entire limb from the pelvic socket. For all other purposes, the surgeon removes the limb at the level of the proximal, one-third of the femur bone.

Before undertaking a limb amputation, the other limbs and the back must be fully evaluated to ensure the dog will have the ability to compensate for the lost limb. If degenerative changes or arthritis in joints of other limbs exist, especially hip joints or back problems, the dog may have problems ambulating postoperatively. In that case, amputation may not be in the dog's best interest. The evaluation should include a thorough physical exam, a gait analysis, a neurological exam, radiographs, and a nuclear bone scan if possible (especially if the amputation is due to a malignant cancer).

A normal healthy dog, young or old, big or small, would be able to easily and smoothly ambulate, run, and play on three limbs. But an arthritic dog or a dog with degenerative changes in its back, young or old, will not adjust as easily and sometimes not at all. Serious consideration of the dog's physical status must occur prior to any amputation. Mentally, dogs immediately adjust to an amputation. They do not appear to "miss" the limb.

The recommended locations of amputation for both the hind and forelimb result in the most aesthetic outcome. If the forelimb is amputated leaving the scapula bone, the muscles associated with the scapula atrophy and the sleek natural body line is interrupted. When amputating a hind limb, the proximal third of the femur is left to cover the groin area which appears to be preferred by owners. Regardless of the location of the lesion (unless it is the toe), the amputations are performed at the locations discussed.

Although at first it may seem radical or excessive to the owner, a dog's amputation cannot be compared to a human amputation. A dog cannot receive and would not use a prosthetic limb. Therefore, any limb portion left remaining would be less aesthetic than no limb, would draw attention to the defect, and, most important, would throw off the dog's balance. It would also most likely become traumatized by normal activity (the end of a stump may get caught on things or get scraped), and dogs frequently chew on the remaining stump (this could be related to the described phenomenon of "ghost pain"). Postoperatively, a snug bandage is placed for three to five days to prevent seroma formation.

The only time that less than the entire limb is removed is if only one or two toes need to be amputated. Then just the toes are amputated. When amputating toes, two rules should be followed in order to maintain limb function:

1. No more than two toes can be removed.
2. At least one of the middle toes must remain.

Limb function may be compromised and the dog could be left with a useless limb if these rules are ignored. Also, when amputating the third digit, the pad must be left to ensure the arterial blood supply is not compromised.

Tail amputation performed for trauma or neurological dysfunction (it also may be required for tail fold pyoderma or perianal fistulas) should be done high to prevent trauma, self-mutilation, or interference with urination and defecation. Postoperatively, a bandage is placed for two to three days, or longer if the dog self-mutilates.

It should be noted, recent studies of cases of perianal fistulas report that a dog with a fistula holds its tail base low, possibly due to cauda equina pain, and surgical correction of the spinal lesion may alleviate the need to perform a tail amputation. The dog may hold its tail in a normal position without pain, allowing fistulas to heal. These studies, however, are inconclusive and are still under investigation.

Excision arthoplasty is indicated when joint pain, usually caused by degenerative changes allowing bone-to-bone contact, occurs. Removal of the joint surface will alleviate pain.

This technique, is generally performed on although not limited to, the coxofemoral (hip) joint. It offers great results in cats and small dogs (total hip implants are not made small enough at this time to be able to fit small animals) who are light and agile enough to compensate.

Surgery involves excision or removal of the head of the femur, the "ball" of the ball and socket joint. This eliminates the painful bone-to-bone contact in the degenerated joint. A fibrous joint forms in its place. This fibrous joint is scar formation and has a limited range of motion. Postoperatively it is important to begin passive and active physical therapy immediately. Normal activity is allowed four to five weeks postoperatively.

In any pet that has undergone excision of the femoral head of the coxofemoral joint, it is crucial to keep its weight down. A dog that has received bilateral femoral head ostectomies (excision) may run with a bunny hop, planting both hind feet together. The dog runs in this manner because the flexion and extension necessary to run cannot be achieved by the limited range of motion of the new fibrous joint, and thus it is accomplished by flexing and extending the thoracolumbar spine.

Salvage procedures exist in everyday prosthetic joint medicine. Hopefully with advances made in prosthetics, transplants may lessen the need for salvage surgeries, but for some situations, such as cancer, they will always exist. When considering a salvage procedure, it is very important that the owner does not place human emotions on the dog.

A qualified surgeon recommends a salvage procedure only when necessary (always get a second opinion). The offending joint or limb is painful and useless to the dog, and it greatly affects the dog's quality of life. Any movement while the dog is awake or even asleep may disrupt the bad leg and cause pain. The dog becomes pain free and much happier postoperatively.

A dog does not appear to have the ability to "miss" the limb, does not "become embarrassed" because it is different or looks strange, and does not "care what other dogs think." It takes a dog a short period of time to adjust to three legs (or an arthrodesed joint), but adjustments occur remarkably fast. (And the dog still has one leg more than humans and we manage okay!) Dogs love their owners in spite of the fact that humans only have two legs, the owner should be able to love the dog with three legs.

FINDING AN ORTHOPEDIC SURGEON

Surgical specialists are available in every state, and your veterinarian should be able to supply you with the name of a specialist in your area. Specialists are boarded by the American College of Veterinary Surgeons (ACVS), whose membership requires post-veterinary formal study, the completion of a surgical residency, and successful completion of written examinations. Carefully assess general practice veterinarians who attempt complicated orthopedic procedures. Although some may be

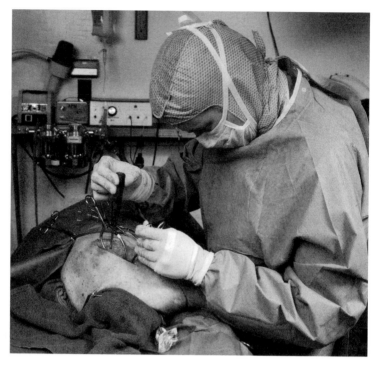

The American College of Veterinary Surgeons confers diplomate status on those who qualify as specialists.

skilled in the procedures, others may lack the experience to provide you with the best possible odds.

Veterinary teaching schools are equipped and staffed to perform orthopedic surgeries, as are many private practices. To locate a qualified surgeon, contact ACVS or a veterinary teaching institution in your area.

American College of Veterinary Surgeons
Alan Lipowitz, DVM,
    Executive Secretary
University of Minnesota
College of Veterinary Medicine
1352 Boyd Ave.
St. Paul, MN 55108

Auburn University
College of Veterinary Medicine
180 Green Hall
Auburn, AL 36849

University of California at Davis
School of Veterinary Medicine
Davis, CA 95616

Colorado State University
College of Veterinary Medicine
and Biomedical Sciences
W102 Anatomy Building
Fort Collins, CO 80523

Cornell University
College of Veterinary Medicine
Ithaca, NY 14853

University of Florida
College of Veterinary Medicine
P.O. Box 100125
Gainesville, FL 32610-0125

University of Illinois
College of Veterinary Medicine
2001 South Lincoln
Urbana, IL 61801

Iowa State University
College of Veterinary Medicine
Ames, IA 50011

Kansas State University
College of Veterinary Medicine
Anderson Hall, Room 9
Manhattan, KS 66506-0117

Louisiana State University
School of Veterinary Medicine
South Stadium Dr.
Baton Rouge, LA 70803-8402

Michigan State University
College of Veterinary Medicine
A-12E East Fee Hall
East Lansing, MI 48824-1316

University of Minnesota
College of Veterinary Medicine
1365 Gortner Ave.
St. Paul, MN 55108

Mississippi State University
College of Veterinary Medicine
Box 9825
Mississippi State, MS 39762

University of Missouri
College of Veterinary Medicine
Columbia, MO 65211

North Carolina State University
College of Veterinary Medicine
4700 Hillsborough St.
Raleigh, NC 27606

Ohio State University
College of Veterinary Medicine
101 Sisson Hall
1900 Coffey Rd.
Columbus, OH 43210

Oklahoma State University
College of Veterinary Medicine
Stillwater, OK 74078-0353

Oregon State University
College of Veterinary Medicine
Magruder Hall 200
Corvallis, OR 97331-4304

University of Pennsylvania
School of Veterinary Medicine
3800 Spruce St.
Philadelphia, PA 19104-6044

Purdue University
School of Veterinary Medicine
Lynn Hall, Room 113
West Lafayette, IN 47907

University of Tennessee
P.O. Box 1071
Knoxville, TN 37901-1071

Texas A & M University
College of Veterinary Medicine
College Station, TX 77843-4461

Tufts University
School of Veterinary Medicine
200 Westboro Rd.
North Grafton, MA 01536

Tuskegee University
School of Veterinary Medicine
Patterson Hall
Tuskegee, AL 36088

Virginia Tech and University of Maryland
Virginia-Maryland Regional
College of Veterinary Medicine
Blacksburg, VA 24061

Washington State University
College of Veterinary Medicine
Pullman, WA 99164-7012

University of Wisconsin
School of Veterinary Medicine
2015 Linden Dr. West
Madison, WI 53706

CHAPTER 17

AT-HOME
POST-SURGICAL CARE

Nursing care for your pet does not end with the animal hospital. Your pet's return home to comfortable surroundings marks a new stage in the recovery period. Having your pet back home is a welcome event, but pet owners must realize that the success of any surgical or medical treatment depends on the aftercare given to the animal. Carefully follow your veterinarian's instructions for your pet's home care.

MEDICATIONS

It is critical that you carefully follow the instructions provided for giving medications to your pet. Dosage and frequency of administration should be noted at discharge and on the label of the medication container.

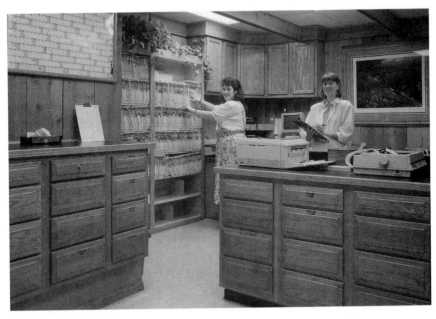

The veterinarian should provide specific instructions for at-home care following any surgery. The discharge process should include instructions, medications, and equipment to follow the doctor's orders.

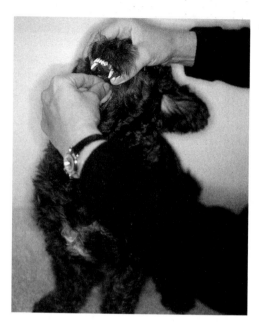

Give all medication as prescribed.
Illustration by Stone Perales

Give all of the medication as prescribed. Even if the pet seems to be feeling better, *continue medicating as prescribed*.

Be sure that the pet swallows and holds down the medication given. To give a pill: Place the pill at the back of the dog or cat's throat, hold the mouth shut, and tilt the head up as you stroke the throat. The pet should swallow the pill without a problem.

Many pets who resist taking medication will accept dosages hidden in treats. A pill disguised in a piece of a hot dog or a roll of cheese can add enjoyment to the act. (However, you must follow diet guidelines prescribed by your veterinarian.)

Administering liquid medication is easily accomplished with the right tools. Don't expect your pet to lick medicine from a spoon. A medicine syringe, which can be supplied by your veterinarian or pharmacy, can be filled to the indicated dosage. Hold your pet and open his or her mouth. Empty the syringe into the back of the mouth cavity, and let your pet swallow. It is possible to stroke the animal's throat to encourage swallowing. Be sure the dog or cat doesn't spit out the medication.

Follow the medication with a tasty treat, if possible. Pets are less likely to spit out or regurgitate the medicine if they want to keep down the treat. If your pet resists the medication, contact the animal hospital for help in handling the situation. Some pets become aggressive when medications are administered. Do not endanger yourself; seek the advice of your veterinarian in handling aggressive pets.

Injections are sometimes given by pet owners. Be sure to follow the instructions given by your veterinarian about dosage and administration. Dispose of supplies responsibly (Return needles to the animal hospital for disposal).

Observe your pet carefully over time, and report any abnormalities to your veterinarian.

CONFINEMENT

Following hospital discharge, many pets must be "kept quiet". When veterinarians give these instructions, they are telling pet owners to keep the pet confined, allowing the pet to rest as much as possible.

A successful surgical procedure or medical treatment can be ruined by a pet who runs loose and damages the area that was just repaired. Many pets, especially dogs who have undergone orthopedic surgeries, are best managed at home by using a crate for confinement, except for short walks on a leash to the toilet area. If owners are unfamiliar with crates, they may initially object to them, but understanding the *dog's perspective* will help. All canines, including dogs, wolves, and foxes, seek a den-like area for security and safety. A dog crate, which is dark, quiet,

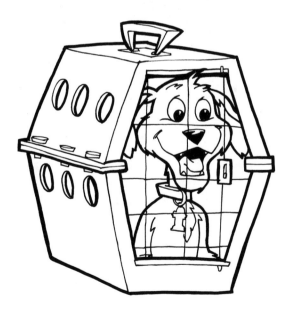

A crate can help you help your dog. This den-like structure prevents dogs from damaging recently repaired joints.   *Illustration by Stone Perales*

and secure, simulates the den that dogs naturally desire, especially when they are injured, sick, or recuperating. Even when they are in good health, dogs view the crate as children view having their own room. In a crate, the dog is protected from nuisances (as wild canines are protected from predators in their dens). No one will tease dogs or disturb them in their dens. A crate is quiet, secluded, and allows the dog to rest without the feeling of being "on duty" to guard and protect the home.

If your veterinarian allows it, you may bring the dog out of the crate for short periods of human interaction, but keep the dog on its leash (even while indoors). Keep the dog tethered to you at all times, and follow your veterinarian's advice for *gradually* returning the dog to normal activities. Also follow your veterinarian's instructions for confining your dog—don't chance reinjury to a repaired limb or stress to a compromised body system.

ELIZABETHAN COLLARS

To keep pets from harming themselves, veterinarians sometimes send pets home with an Elizabethan collar, a plastic device that prohibits pets from licking various areas of their bodies. The collar (which is

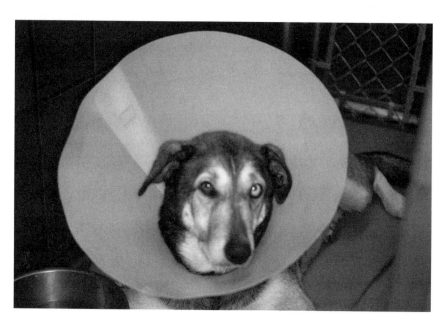

Pets can eat, drink, and perform regular activities while wearing an Elizabethan collar.

named after the elaborate, wide collars that appeared on the dresses of women of leisure in the Elizabethan period) prevents pets from tearing out stitches, removing or damaging bandages, irritating sensitive skin, and infecting incision sites. Pets can eat, drink, and perform regular activities while wearing the collars. Do not remove the collar, even at night, or the pet could quickly injure itself. Pets can learn to walk up stairs, get through doorways, and sleep comfortably while wearing these collars. For your pet's sake, keep the collar on as prescribed by the veterinarian.

BANDAGING

Your veterinarian should provide you with instructions for cleaning wounds and changing bandages. Hot or cold compresses (towels soaked in water and placed on the wound site) may be advised. Keeping the bandaged area clean and dry is critical to healing, and regular bandage changing is part of the hygiene ritual. Medications and ointments should be administered as directed by the veterinarian.

Some bandages can be changed at home, others may need the attention of the veterinary hospital personnel. Adhere to the recommended bandaging schedule, and report any abnormalities to your veterinarian.

Regularly observe surgery or abrasion sites, and check for red, inflamed areas. Discharge at the incision line should be reported to your veterinarian.

WHEN TO CALL THE VETERINARIAN

Expect a convalescing pet to sleep more, eat a little less, and lack some energy, but extreme variation should be reported to the veterinarian immediately.

Furthermore, any of the following signs could indicate an emergency and should be reported without delay:

- Shortness of breath
- Open wounds
- Temperatures over 105 degrees Fahrenheit
- Profuse bleeding
- Frequent urination
- Difficulty urinating or defecating
- Crying

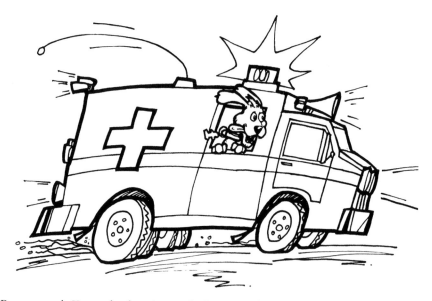

Be prepared. Know the location and phone number of your nearest veterinary emergency clinic.   *Illustration by Stone Perales*

- Uncontrollable panting

- Vomiting

- Diarrhea

- Failure to eat

- Straining to walk

Surgery provides an opportunity to return your dog to an active lifestyle. Post-surgical care is critical to the success of the surgery and depends on you observing the instructions for recuperation.

ROUTINE CARE

Maintaining a good preventive care program is essential for the well-being of your pet. Parasite control, vaccinations, dental care, and routine examinations should be scheduled with your regular veterinarian. Keep these programs on schedule to ensure that your pet maintains good health.

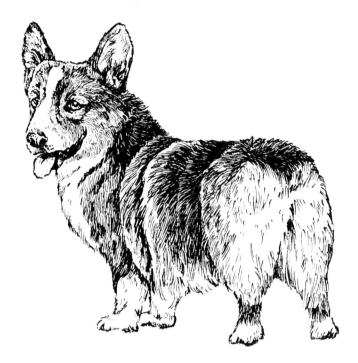

Beware of dogs that look "ready to rumble." Limit physical exercise if your veterinarian advises doing so.   *Illustration by Chris Hoy*

EMERGENCIES

Know the location and operating hours of your nearest emergency-care
animal hospital. Post the phone number in a convenient place in your
house, such as on the refrigerator. Keep calm in an emergency and
contact the emergency clinic for instructions on caring for your pet.

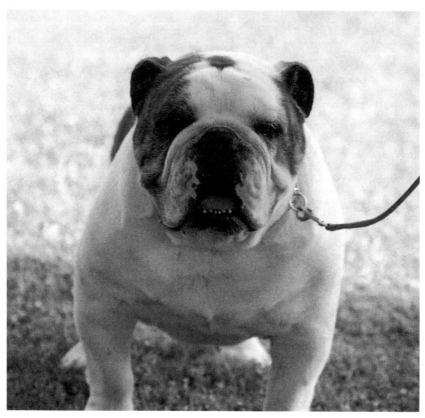

A dog's health and happiness depend on the owner's dedication to fulfilling the animal's needs. Practice preventive medicine, and don't ignore signs of pain or illness.

CHAPTER 18

ETHICAL
CONSIDERATIONS

Orthopedic illnesses are painful for those stricken with the various conditions. At best, the disease may limit activity or cause occasional pain. At worst, crippling, debilitating pain and the inability to bear weight renders the victim unable to perform normal daily activities, such as walking through the house, defecating without support, or sleeping comfortably through the night.

It is simply unconscionable to ignore these diseases. While minor injuries can repair without medical intervention, chronic or severe conditions require a veterinarian's skills to return the dog to an active lifestyle free from pain. Hoping the signs will just go away won't change a dog's physical condition, and delay in seeking help may cause a disease to progress or may rob the dog of the chance to mend to full potential. Delays always make the dog endure prolonged pain and suffering, which sometimes can be avoided with pharmaceutical, physical therapy, or surgical treatment.

Pet ownership is a privilege and a responsibility. Accepting responsibility for a dog extends beyond feeding and flea control. Health care for pets involves routine medical care as well as planning for the unexpected. Although medical costs can be burdensome, most agree that a pet's well-being justifies the expense. Although veterinarians strive to keep medical costs affordable, the cost of providing veterinary services is quite expensive, and pet owners must absorb the costs of caring for their pets.

Pet care costs exceed the price of pet purchase. However, the benefits of pet ownership have proven to more than compensate for the costs incurred. "Investing" in pets is among the most conservative of expenditures. The paybacks received from a loyal dog include unconditional companionship, undying affection, and comfort in times of sorrow. Dogs have been know to lift spirits and lower blood pressure. The value of owning a dog increases as pet owners commit increased time and emotion to the relationship they share with their dogs.

Honoring the sanctity of the human/animal bond requires that we acknowledge our pets' needs and make choices with their best interests in mind. Pet owners, breeders, and veterinarians should examine their consciences each time they make a decision regarding an orthopedic disease found in dogs. Each should consider the aspects that pertain to their part in controlling, preventing, and treating disease and trauma. Introspection can begin by asking the following questions:

THE PET OWNER

1. Have I protected my dog from the threat of injury by securing the dog in a safe environment? Are my fences solid and is the dog kept on a leash when walked? Have we completed basic Obedience training, and does my dog respond to Come, Stay, and Down? Obeying these commands could save a dog's life and protect it from injury.
2. Have I spayed or neutered my pet? Just because I love my dog doesn't mean the dog should reproduce. Unless breeders have thoroughly researched the pedigrees of their dogs, along with the pedigrees of the dogs they breed with, they may be creating dogs with genetically linked diseases, such as hip dysplasia or wobblers syndrome. Commitment to producing sound puppies requires an investment of time and money. Usually breeders with working, show, or Obedience lines have the commitment to thoroughly

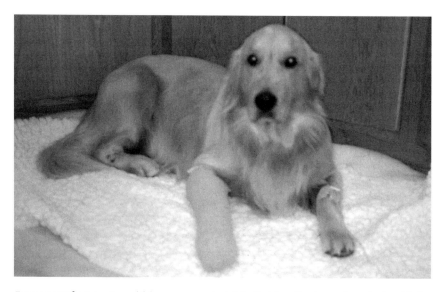

Proper confinement could have prevented this Golden Retriever from being hit by a car.

Popular breeds, such as this Cocker Spaniel, often suffer from their appeal. People can be tempted to breed their dogs because they know there is a market for puppies. Before breeding, responsible breeders evaluate a dog's genetic composition, both from personal knowledge and medical testing, rather than just responding to a demand for puppies.

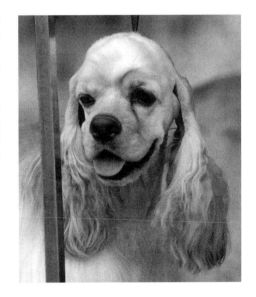

research pedigrees (knowing not just the names of dogs in the family tree, but also the dogs' physical histories, which is necessary for making breeding decisions).

3. Have I maintained ongoing physical care for my dog? Puppy health-care programs and annual physical examinations allow veterinarians to thoroughly assess a dog's health, even before seeing signs of disease or illness. Early detection often provides opportunities to treat disease before irreversible damage has been done. Furthermore, when your veterinarian is familiar with what is "normal" for your dog, he or she will be better able to notice when your dog is not right.

4. Have I provided for my pet's needs? Dogs require veterinary care, *especially* in their senior years. Extending quality and length of life may depend upon specialized veterinary care.

THE BREEDER

1. Is this dog of the quality to be bred? Breeders should keep excellent health records and compare findings with others in their breed. Honest conversations can go far to enhance a breed's overall health profile. Dishonest or negligent breeding produces problems in dogs that can infiltrate the breed and take generations to overcome.

2. Have I exhausted all avenues for critiquing my dogs' breeding potential? Every stud dog and brood bitch should be thoroughly examined

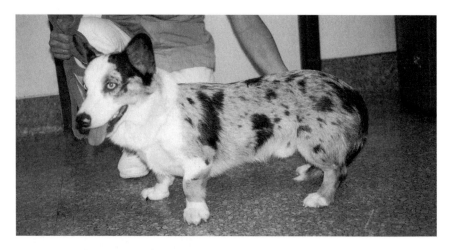

Breeders should become familiar with the diseases that threaten their breeds. Chondrodysplastic (short-legged) dogs, such as the two Corgi breeds, can be predisposed to disk disease. Responsible breeders monitor the dogs in their lines and make breeding decisions to avoid producing disease in their puppies.

for detectable congenital diseases. All dogs, especially large dogs, should be x-rayed for evidence of hip dysplasia. OFA and PennHIP® studies should confirm a breeder's speculation that a dog's hips are sound. Studies of elbows, knees, and backs also prove valuable. Nonorthopedic concerns, such as progressive retinal atrophy, von Willebrand's disease, and thyroid abnormalities should also be screened in those breeds affected by the conditions.

3. Am I kennel blind? *Not all dogs should be bred.* Even dogs with superlative pedigrees may not live up to expectations. Think with your head, not just your heart.
4. Am I sharing my knowledge? Serve as a mentor to your puppy buyers. Advise them of your concerns and your pleasure in seeing well-bred dogs mature. Help friends and relatives make good decisions about their dogs.

THE VETERINARIAN

1. Have I spent enough time with my clients to perform a thorough examination? Look for things you don't expect to find.
2. Have I advised clients in the best interest of the dog, rather than trying to tell people what they want to hear? Of course diplomacy is a requirement when practicing medicine of any type, but sometimes difficult discussions must take place.

A solid pet owner/veterinarian relationship is the key to establishing the groundwork for a wonderful pet-owning experience.

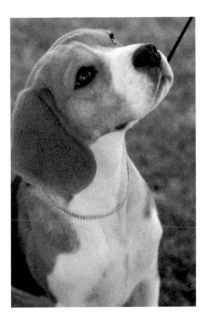

3. Have I provided clients with *all* options available for treating their pets, not just the options I can perform in my clinic? Veterinarians should avoid making financial or ethical decisions for pet owners, but rather should serve as sources of information and consultation. Many pet owners opt to secure extensive medical care for pets they adore.
4. Have I been honest in my assessment of a condition? Sometimes the truth hurts, but in the long run false hopes crash down harder.

Emotions sometimes cloud our judgment capabilities. We need logic and true compassion to prevent tragedies from occurring. We should do everything in our power to provide our dogs with the best possible quality of life, and we should do everything to avoid creating (through breeding and advising) hardships for other people and animals to endure.

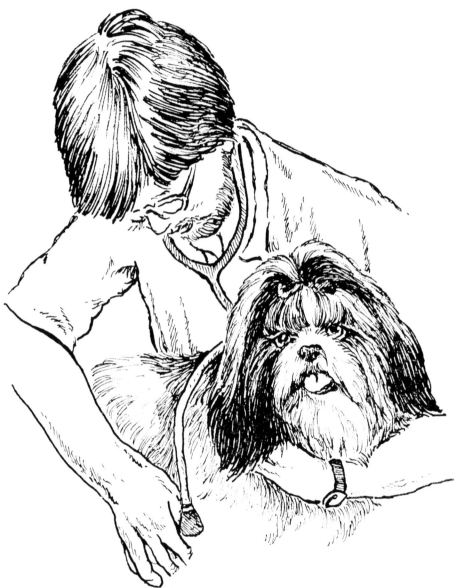

Pets and people benefit from the curiosity and dedication of scientific minds.

Illustration by Chris Hoy

CHAPTER 19

SCIENTIFIC
ADVANCEMENTS

Scientific, medical, and technological advances improve medicine on a daily basis. Advances in human medicine benefit dogs and cats, just as work with dogs and cats can help further human medical practices. Orthopedics certainly is a field where progressive, ongoing work to improve procedures such as total hip replacement implants, artificial prostheses, and bone and nerve regeneration benefits not only humans, but animals as well.

TOTAL HIP REPLACEMENT

Until recently, the total hip replacement implant was a steel fixed-head system. The head and stem were a single unit, thus the neck length of the implant could not be selected to accommodate the various sizes of adult dogs. This limited accessibility to usable parts limited the success of the procedure for dogs that did not "fit the mold."

A newly designed modular system has recently been made available to veterinary surgeons. The system features separate stem and head implants. This modular system has several advantages over the old, fixed system. First, it allows different neck lengths (three choices) dependent on the size and angle appropriate for the dog. A head and neck locking system, capable of handling rotation and distraction loads, makes the system even more desirable. The stem offers five sizes, and four acetabular cup sizes are available. The variation available with the modular system achieves greater flexibility in the size of the patient (14 kg—no upper limit) and allows the surgeon to accommodate the patient's needs in surgery. The cup is composed of high-density polyethylene, and the head and stem are composed of cobalt-chrome (older implants were made of steel or titanium).

The total hip implants are secured in place with bone cement, polymethyl methacrylate (PMMA). Although relatively infrequent, a complication noted with PMMA involves sciatic nerve damage (a temporary condition) resulting from heat that is released when the PMMA hardens.

Surgeons have been working with a cementless prosthesis that is technically more difficult to implant than the traditional cemented device. However, the new prosthesis may be associated with fewer complications and may be more secure once in place. This prosthesis is not yet commercially available, but the testing looks very promising.

For dogs with hip instability, but without secondary osteoarthosis, a new procedure, biocompatible osteoconductive polymer (BOP) shelf arthroplasty, was thought to show promise. This procedure uses a biocompatible graft to extend (or shelf) the rim of a shallow acetabulum. It was hoped the BOP substance would actually induce new bone growth. Data on this procedure has not been promising; the BOP substance does not appear to promote growth and may hinder new bone growth. Although developed to enhance joint stability, the loading forces on the articular cartilage remain abnormal, therefore the secondary osteoarthritis continues. For these reasons, this procedure (unless redesigned) will most likely not be pursued.

In veterinary medicine the only widely accepted prosthesis is for the hip joint. The hip joint is a ball and socket joint and the easiest joint to duplicate. Arthroplasty using joint implants designed for humans may become more commonplace. A human wrist prosthesis, available in 10 sizes, will fit many cat and dog joints. Smaller joints may be replaced with finger joint implants. Although wrist prostheses have successfully replaced arthritic and deformed elbow joints in the dog, these have been too few to be conclusive yet. Further studies will hopefully be able to report successful procedures available to every patient.

Advancements in veterinary medicine result from a collaborative effort of many people. University and industrial scientists, practicing health professionals, and patients who are willing to explore new concepts enable discoveries to be made. Contributions come from many unexpected sources. For example, scientific studies conducted by the space program may result in advancements in the treatment of spinal injuries. The effects of weightlessness and the shock of reentry into our atmosphere may trigger a nerve response that regenerates. Who knows what the future will bring, but each day we learn something new and valuable.

GLOSSARY

Abduction The movement of a part away from the median plane. For a digit, the drawing away from the axis of the limb; for a limb, the drawing away from the body.

Acetabulum The cup-shaped socket of the hip joint that houses the head of the femur. Used as an indicator of proper laxity in the canine hip joint and in radiographic assessment for hip dysplasia.

Achilles tendon The common group of tendons that inserts on the heel near the point of the hock.

Acromion The prominence at the far end of the spine of the scapula. (Adj. **acromial**)

Actinomycin A family of antibiotics from various species of streptomyces, which are active against bacteria and funguses.

Adduction Drawing a limb toward the body. The movement of a part toward the median plane.

Allograft A graft between individuals of the same species, but of different genotypes (i.e., two unrelated dogs).

Aminoglycosides Any of a group of bacterial antibiotics derived from various species of streptomyces (with sugars) that interfere with the function of bacterial ribosomes.

Amputation The removal of a limb or other appendage or outgrowth of the body. The most common indication for amputation of a limb is severe trauma. Other indications may include malignancy, neoplasia, and infection.

Analgesia Absence of sensibility to pain, particularly the relief of pain, without loss of consciousness.

Anastomosis 1. Communication between two tubular organs. 2. Surgical, traumatic, or pathological formation of a connection between two normally distinct structures. (Adj. anastomotic)

Anconal, anconeal Pertaining to the elbow.

Anconeal process The projection of the ulna near the back of the humerus, which develops as a separate ossification center in some dogs.

Ankle A human anatomical term often applied to dogs when referring to the hock joint.

Ankylo   Word element [Greek]. Bent, crooked, in the form of a loop, adhesion, fixed.

Ankylosis   Abnormal immobility and consolidation of a joint (Adj. ankylotic)

Antebrachiocarpal   Pertaining to the joint between the forearm and the carpus. Called also proximal carpal or radiocarpal joint.

Antibiotic   1. Destructive of life. 2. A chemical produced by a microorganism that has the capacity (in dilute solutions) to kill (biocidal activity) or inhibit the growth (biostatic activity) of microorganisms. Antibiotics that are *not* toxic to the host are used as chemotheraputic agents in the treatment of infectious diseases.

Anticoagulant   1. Preventing the coagulation of blood. 2. Any substance that suppresses, delays, or nullifies coagulation of blood. There is limited therapeutic use for anticoagulants in animals; their importance is in the collection of blood for testing and for transfusion.

Arthralgia   Pain in a joint.

Arthritis   Inflammation of a joint.

Arthrocentesis   Sterile puncture of a joint cavity for aspiration of fluid, usually for diagnostic purposes.

Arthrochondritis   Inflammation of the cartilage of a joint.

Arthrodesis   Surgical fusion of a joint.

Arthrolysis   Operative loosening of adhesions in a joint.

Arthrometer   An instrument for assessing the angles of joint movements (also called a goniometer).

Arthropathy   Any joint disease.

Articular   Pertaining to a joint.

Aspirin   A common drug generally used to relieve pain and reduce fever. Can be toxic in normal doses. The cat is particularly susceptible. Clinical signs of toxicity are hemorrhagic gastritis, hyperexcitability, and metabolic acidosis. When given to dogs, aspirin is recommended to have an enteric coating.

Autograft   A graft transferred from one part of the patient's body to another.

Avulsion   The tearing away of a structure or part.

Axial   1. The central line of the body, or any of its parts, around which the structure moves. 2. Pertinent to, or deriving from, the axis bone of the vertebral column.

Bacterial   Pertaining to or caused by bacteria.

Bandage   1. A strip or roll of gauze or other material for wrapping or binding any part of the body. 2. Cover by wrapping with such material. Bandages may be used to stop the flow of blood, to provide a safeguard against contamination, or to hold a medicated dressing in place. They may also be used to hold a splint in position or immobilize an injured part of the body to prevent further injury and to facilitate healing.

Biceps   A muscle having two heads. There is a biceps muscle in both the forelimbs and the hind limbs.

Biomechanics   The application of mechanical laws to living structures.

Biopsy   Removal and examination, usually microscopic, of tissue from the living body. Biopsies are usually done to determine whether a tumor is malignant or benign; however, a biopsy may be a useful diagnostic tool in other disease processes, such as infections.

Blood chemistry   Also called **serum chemistry.** Measurement of chemical enzymes and constituents present in the blood. Used to rule out or confirm a differential diagnosis.

Bone   1. The hard, rigid form of connective tissue constituting most of the skeleton of most vertebrates and composed chiefly of an organic component of collagenous matrix, cells, and a mineral component of calcium phosphate and other salts. 2. Any distinct piece of the skeleton of the body. 3. Describes conformation, substance, thickness, and quality of bone structure in an animal; e.g., an animal with good bone.

Bone cysts   A discrete, grossly visible cavity filled with fluid and often lined by a membrane. It may be a single cavity (unicameral), be located under cartilage (subchondral), be filled with blood (aneurysmal), or contain epidermal cells (epidermoid).

Bone grafts   The transfer of a piece of bone, usually for fracture repair or reconstructive surgery. Various types of bone grafts are identified, depending on their source and treatment (e.g., cortical, autograft, allograft, cancellous, xenograft, isograft).

Brachium   The arm, specifically from the shoulder to the elbow; also called thoracic limb.

Calcaneus   The largest tarsal bone; it forms the heel.

Calcium   Calcium is the most abundant mineral in the body. In combination with phosphorus, it forms calcium phosphate, the dense, hard material of the bones and teeth. It is an important element in intracellular and extracellular fluid and is essential to the normal clotting of blood, the maintenance of a normal heartbeat, and the initiation of neuromuscular and metabolic activities.

Calcium homeostasis   Maintenance of normal calcium metabolism by the combined effects of adequate food intake, renal excretion, parathyroid hormone involvement, plasma protein binding, and deposition in tissues.

Callus   1. Localized hyperplasia of the horny layer of the epidermis due to pressure or friction. In dogs, these often form over pressure points, such as the elbow, hock, and (in some breeds) the sternum, particularly if the animal is sleeping on a hard surface. 2. An unorganized network of woven bone formed about the ends of a broken bone, absorbed as repair is completed (provisional callus) and ultimately replaced by true bone (definitive callus).

Canaliculi bone Branching tubular passages radiating like wheel spokes from each bone lacuna to connect with similar structures and with the Haversian canal (longitudinal canals within the bone).

Carpal Pertaining to the wrist (carpus).

Cartilage A specialized, gristly connective tissue present in both mature animals and embryos providing a model in which most of the bones develop. Constituting an important part of the organism's growth mechanism, the three most important types are hyaline cartilage, elastic cartilage, and fibrocartilage. Also a general term for a mass of such tissue in a particular site in the body.

Cast 1. A positive copy of an object e.g., a mold of a hollow organ formed of effused plastic matter and extruded from the body. 2. A stiff dressing, or casing, usually made of plaster of paris used to immobilize body parts. More modern, lightweight casts are made of polyurethane resins.

Catheter A tubular, flexible instrument for withdrawal of fluids from (or introduction of fluids into) a body cavity, vein, or artery.

Caudal The direction toward the animal's tail.

Cervical Pertaining to the neck or to the cervix.

Chondroblasts An immature, cartilage-producing cell.

Chondrocalcinosis Deposits of calcium salts in the joint cartilage.

Chondroclasts A giant cell believed to be concerned in absorption of cartilage.

Chondrocyte A mature cartilage cell embedded in a lacuna within the cartilage matrix.

Collateral 1. Secondary or accessory; not direct or immediate. 2. A side branch, as of a blood vessel or nerve.

Compaction Packing together, as in twin births when both fetuses engage the pelvis at the same time, in prolonged constipation in dogs, and in compaction of endochondral bone, as a part of normal bone modeling.

Compression 1. The act of pressing upon or together; the state of being pressed together. A specific example is compression plating in fracture repair. 2. In embryology, the shortening or omission of certain developmental stages.

Condyles A rounded projection on a bone, usually for articulation with another bone; a knuckle.

Coombs test Laboratory test that reveals certain antigen-antibody reactions, used in differentiating between various types of hemolytic anemias, for determining minor blood types, and for testing for alloimmune hemolytic disease of the newborn. Also called antiglobulin tests.

Coronoid process A part of the elbow joint. A beak-like projection on either side of the trochlear notch of the ulna.

Cortex The outer layer of an organ or structure, such as bone or a kidney.

Cortical Pertaining to or emanating from a cortex or outer layer of a structure.

Corticosteroids Hormones produced by the adrenal cortex; they may also be of a synthetic origin, divided into glucocorticoids, mineralocorticoids, and androgens.

Coxa valga Deformity of the hip joint changing the angle of the femur.

Coxofemoral joint Pertaining to the hip.

Cranial The direction toward the animal's head.

Cranial drawer movement The drawer sign is abnormal forward movement of the tibia relative to the femur which is held in a stable position. (from pg. 117)

Craniomandibular osteopathy (CMO) An hereditary disorder; a symmetrical bony enlargement of the mandible.

Creep A barrier with small openings often used for feeding purposes to allow young animals access to the feed.

Crepitus A crackling sound or sensation; grating ends of bone in a fracture or abnormal joint.

Cruciate ligament A ligament positioned in a crisscross formation, associated with the stifle joint; it may become torn or ruptured, causing lameness.

Cutaneous Pertaining to the skin.

Cyclophosphamide A neoplastic suppressant used to treat abnormal cell development, whether malignant or benign.

Cytokines Biologic proteins; an important part of the cell-mediated immune reaction.

Cytological examination The study of cell structure, function, and pathology, usually from a fluid within the body.

Debridement The removal of contaminated, damaged, or dead tissue from an injured or infected lesion.

Decompression The return to a normal pressure; i.e., spinal cord decompression or gastric decompression.

Decortication Removal of the cortical surface of an organ or structure.

Deep pain A response that may or may not be elicited during a neurological examination for the conscious perception of pain.

Deformation An alteration of normal shape or structure.

Degenerative Deterioration or a less functional form, as in degenerative joint disease.

Dehiscence The separation of the layers of a surgical incision.

Delayed union Slower than normal or prolonged time for healing, as in orthopedic or wound healing.

Dewclaw The rudimentary first digit (or thumb) of the dog; A non-weight bearing digit. If removed, commonly done at three days of age to prevent future injury.

Dexamethasone   A synthetic glucocorticoid used as an anti-inflammatory medication.

Diagnosis   A name given to a disease syndrome; an analysis leading to treatment, prescription, and prognosis.

Diaphysis   The central region of the bone (bone shaft), either between the ends or extremities.

Digital extensor   A muscle or ligament that extends the digit (i.e., the toe).

Discospondylitis   A destructive, inflammatory process involving the intervertebral disks.

Disk ruptures   Intervertebral disk pad dislocation by extrusion or protrusion between two vertebrae affecting the spinal cord.

Dislocations   Displacement of a bone from a joint.

Displacement   Movement to an abnormal location or position.

Distal   The direction *away from* the main portion of a structure. When describing the limbs, this would be the paws.

Distraction   The separation of joint surfaces without rupture or displacement.

Dorsal   The portion of the body near the back surface from the head following the spinal cord to the tail.

Dynamic   Orthopedic compression plates that exhibit a force to the bone; pertaining to force.

Dysplasia   Abnormal development.

Eburnated bone   Bone conversion to a hard ivory-like mass.

Ectrodactyly   The congenital absence of a complete or portion of a digit.

Effusions   Fluid that has escaped into another structure.

Ehmer sling   A style of bandage that holds the hind leg in a flexed, non-weight bearing position.

Ehrlichia canis   Causes canine ehrlichiosis, an intracellular parasite.

Ehrlichiosis   A rickettsial disease transmitted by an infected brown dog tick.

Elbow   Lower forelimb; a flexible hinge joint.

Elizabethan collar (restraint)   A cone-shaped device, similar in form to collar fashions during the Elizabethan era, used to prevent the dog's mouth access to other body areas.

Endochondral ossification   Process by which hyaline cartilage is resorbed and replaced by bone.

Endosteum   Osteoblastic lining of the osteons and cortical bone facing the marrow cavity.

Epiphysis   The end of the bone separated by the physial plates in growing animals.

Erosion   Wearing away and loss of substance, often of bone surface.

Excision   Removal of an organ or structure by surgical means.

Extension   Joint angulation is increased; the motion resulting in limb, digit, and back straightening.

External   Situated or occurring on or near the outside.

Fascia lata   A band (layer)of fibrous tissue of the thigh.

Fasciotomy   Incision of a fascia (layer) structure.

Fatigue   Tiredness; related to muscular overexertion.

Femoral   Pertaining to the femur, thigh, or upper portion of the rear leg.

Femoral Head   The "ball" or end of the femur that makes up the part of the hip joint positioned into the acetabular rim or "socket."

Femur   The thigh bone, extending from pelvis (hip) to stifle (knee).

Fiberglass   Material used to form a cast to support a fractured limb; it is lightweight, strong, and quick to "set."

Fibrillation   Small, local, involuntary muscular contractions, usually associated with the heart.

Fibroblasts   Immature connective tissue; can develop into chondroblasts, collagenoblasts, or osteoblasts.

Fibrocartilage   Cartilage made from thick collagenous bundles.

Fibrosarcoma   A sarcoma (cancerous tumor) arising from collagen-producing fibroblasts; can occur in many organs.

Fibrosis   Formation of fibrous tissue.

Fibula   The lateral (outer) bone of the two bones that comprise the lower end of the hind leg, from stifle to hock.

Fixation   Holding or suturing into a fixed position.

Flexion   A bending motion. Joint angulation is reduced, resulting in limb retraction, digits bending, and the back arching.

Flexor response (reflex)   A spinal reflex, usually in response to pain, resulting in flexion or withdrawal of the leg or limb.

Fluid replacement (therapy)   Used to treat fluid loss caused by disease, restricted intake, or fluid excretion.

Fracture   Breaking of a part, particularly bone; different types of fractures may occur from various forces.

Fragmented coronoid process   A developmental lesion of the elbow; also called elbow dysplasia.

Frontal bone   Paired bones making up the upper part of the face/forehead.

Front limb   The forelimb, equivalent to the arms in humans.

Gait   A manner or style of locomotion; may include the walk, trot, or run.

Glycosaminoglycan   Carbohydrates contain these amino sugars; synthetic polysulfated glycosaminoglycans can be administered to increase joint fluid viscosity.

Graft   Tissue or organ implantation to replace damaged or missing tissue, particularly of bone.

Growth   Progressive increase in size; process of physical development.

Head bob   Action observed at slow gait when an abnormal transfer of weight due to lameness causes head to change elevation with movement.

Heat therapy   Hyperthermia application of heat for physical therapy

Hematoma   A localized collection of extravasated blood in an organ, space, or tissue; can occur almost anywhere on the body.

Hematuria   Discharge of blood in urine.

Hind limb   The rear limb or back leg of the dog.

Hip dislocation   A dislocation of the hip joint; the dog is unable to bear full weight on that limb.

Hip dysplasia   A lax joint, a predisposition for which is genetically inherited; lameness may eventually be present.

Hip joint   The ball and socket joint of the pelvis and femur.

Hip prosthesis   A synthetic replacement of the femoral head and acetabular cup.

Hip replacement   A replacement of the femoral head and acetabulum with a prosthesis that is cemented into the bone.

Histological   The structure, composition, and function of tissues.

Histopathological   Determination of the cause of changes from normal structure, composition, and function of tissue.

Hobbles   Straps placed around the carpal joint (wrists) to restrict movement.

Hock   The ankle joint or tarsal joint.

Humeral   Of or pertaining to the humerus.

Humerus   The bone of the upper forelimb, from shoulder to elbow.

Hydrotherapy   External use of water to treat disease or injury, as in a whirlpool bath or swim therapy.

Hyperemia   An excess of blood in a part of the body.

Hyperextension   Extension of a limb beyond its normal limit.

Hyperparathyroidism   Abnormally increased activity of the parathyroid gland; can lead to calcium imbalance causing kidney stones, osteoporosis, or hypercalcemia.

Hyperplasia   Abnormal increase in the volume of a tissue or organ due to the growth of new normal cells.

Hyperthermia   Increased body temperature; heat therapy.

Hypertrophy   Increase in volume of a tissue or organ caused by the enlargement of existing cells.

Hypoplasia   The incomplete development or underdevelopment of an organ or tissue.

Hypovolemic shock   Shock caused by severe blood loss or dehydration.

Idiopathic   Without known cause; usually referring to a disease condition that may be self-originated.

Ilial shaft (or spine)   The portion of the ilium that is cut and repositioned to an improved angle for the pelvic osteotomy, one treatment for canine hip dysplasia.

Ilium   The large spoon- or wing-shaped bone at the cranial end of the pelvis.

Immobilization   Making something or a body part incapable of movement.

Immune system   The primary and secondary lymph organs that form antibodies.

Immune-mediated arthritis   A noninfectious joint disease involving the immune mechanisms.

Implants   To insert or to graft a material into the body i.e., carbon fibre, metal, plastic, hormone, or electronic signal.

Infection   The invasion and multiplication of microorganisms in body tissues; may be due to local injury, toxins, or antigen-antibody response.

Inflammation   A localized response to protect an area of injured tissue and that serves to wall off the injured area from normal tissue; signified by heat, redness, swelling, pain, and loss of function.

Injury   To harm, hurt, or wound; usually caused by an outside force.

Inorganic   A substance that does not contain carbon as a compound.

Intercondylar fracture   A fracture between two condyles, as in the stifle joint.

Internal fixation   Immobilization of fractured bones by internal means; the use of intramedullary pins, screws, or a compression plate and screws.

Intertrochanteric   The area between the greater and lesser trochanter of the femur; the tubers at the proximal (near) end of the femur.

Intervertebral disk   The pad of fibrocartilage between two vertebrae.

Intra-articular fractures   A fracture within a joint.

Ischium   The tail-end (not the tail itself), dorsal portion of the pelvic hip bone; one of the areas surgically cut to reposition the angle in treating canine hip dysplasia.

Joint   The site of the joining of two or more bones; provides mobility, flexibility, and an area for growth.

Joint capsule   Provides stability, nutrition, lubrication, and debris disposal for the joints.

Joint disease   May include arthritis, arthropathy, ankylosis, or degenerative joint disease.

Joint disorders   A derangement or abnormality to joint function; may or may not include disease.

Joint fluid   Produced by synovial membrane; a viscous, transparent, straw-colored fluid that lubricates and provides nutrients to joint tissues.

Joint fracture   May occur in combination with dislocation of the hip and femoral neck fracture; commonly resulting from traffic accidents.

Joint laxity   Abnormal looseness or excessive movement in a joint. Laxity has been shown to be a primary factor for developing degenerative joint disease (DJD).

Joint lubrication   Provided by fluid produced in the synovial membrane.

Kinetic energy   Energy or heat producing or produced by motion.

Kinking of tendons   An abnormal shortening of muscle tissue; can be caused by fibrosis of tissues supporting the muscles; may occur in contracture secondary to casting or splinting.

Kirschner   A German surgeon, Martin Kirschner, for whom surgical equipment is named.

Kirschner apparatus   External skeletal fixation device that provides rigid fixation and controlled stress across a healing fracture.

Kirschner pins   Pins that are available in different sizes to be used with connecting bars for external skeletal fixation.

Klebsiella   A gram-negative bacteria.

Laceration   A wound produced by the tearing of body tissue.

Lamellar bone   Bone matrix deposited in an orderly manner so that the collagen fibers form parallel, microscopic layers. All normal bone of the mature skeleton is lamellar.

Lameness   The state of being lame; deviation from a normal gait.

Laminectomy   Surgical excision of the dorsal arch of a vertebra, performed to reduce compression on the spinal cord by an intervertebral disk.

Lateral   A position away from the midline of the body, or pertaining to the side of the structure.

Legg-Calves Perthes disease   An idiopathic necrosis and lysis of the femoral head.

Leukocytosis   A transient increase in the number of leukocytes in the blood.

Leukopenia   Reduction in the number of leukocytes in the blood.

Ligament   A band of fibrous tissue connecting bones or cartilage; serves to support and strengthen joints. (Adj. ligamentous)

Limb   One of the paired appendages (a leg or arm) used in locomotion.

Linear   In a line.

Lumbar   Pertaining to the loins; lumbar vertebrae are located between the thorax and sacrum.

Luxation   Dislocation.

Lyme disease   An acute, recurrent, polyarthritis caused by a spirochete, Borrelia burgdorferi, transmitted by a brown deer tick.

Lymph nodes An accumulation of lymphoid tissue organized as a lymphoid organ; serves as a defense mechanism, sometimes called a lymph gland.

Magnetic resonance imaging An imaging modality that can demonstrate cross sections of a body part by the realignment of hydrogen ions in cellular structure. Increasingly used in veterinary applications.

Malleolus A rounded process on the distal end of the fibula or tibia.

Malunion Incorrect anatomical alignment or union of fracture fragments.

Mandible The bone forming the lower jaw.

Mandibulectomy The surgical removal of part or all of the mandible.

Marrow Bone marrow; organic material in the center or cavity of bone that produces blood cells.

Massage Therapeutic stroking or kneading of the body or part.

Matrix Collagen and ground substance of bone; bone tissue minus minerals and cells.

Maxilla The bones that form the upper jaw.

Medial Pertains to the center or midline of the body when viewed vertically from head to tail.

Meniscal injury An injury to the meniscus causing instability to the stifle joint, usually with cranial cruciate ligament damage.

Meniscectomy Surgical removal of the meniscus.

Meniscocapsular ligaments The ligaments that attach the menisci to the tibia and fibula.

Meniscotibial ligaments The two ligaments that attach each meniscus to the tibia.

Meniscus The crescent-shaped fibrocartilage pad of the stifle (knee) joint.

Metacarpals The bones comprising the paw of the front limb between the carpus (wrist) and the digits (toes).

Metaphyseal trabeculae The supporting structure of "mesh" that is filled with bone marrow, located in the metaphyseal area.

Metaphysis The wider portion of the end of the shaft of a long bone.

Metastasis The transfer of disease (such as a malignant tumor) from one organ or portion of the body to another.

Metatarsus The bones comprising the paw of the rear limb between the tarsus and digits.

Methylmethacrylate A bone cement that is used in orthopedic repair for spinal conditions or fractures of a limb.

Methylprednisolone A corticosteroid; it has anti-inflammatory action.

Microfracture An extremely small fracture.

Mineralization The addition of mineral matter to the body, especially of the skeleton.

Modeling A simulation or copy of a naturally occurring structure.

Monostotic bone cysts A cyst that forms within a single bone.

Muscle An organ composed of bundles of fibers having the power to contract and thereby produce movement.

Musculoskeletal Pertaining to muscle and skeleton.

Myectomy Excision or cutting of a muscle.

Myelography Radiography of the spinal cord after a contrast agent has been injected into the subarachnoid space.

Myopathy Any disease of a muscle; more commonly describing muscle degeneration or weakness.

Myotomy Cutting of a muscle or muscular tissue.

Nail length An observation made of the toe nails during an orthopedic/neurological examination.

Naproxen A nonsteroidal, anti-inflammatory (NSAID) agent; may cause gastric ulcers in dogs.

Neck The elongated portion of the femur leading to the femoral head.

Necrosis Cell death caused by enzyme degradation.

Neoplasia The formation of a tumor; a new or abnormal growth.

Nerve Conveys impulses between the central nervous system and a part of the body.

Neurofibroma A tumor of peripheral nerves.

Neurological Pertaining to or emanating from the nervous system.

Nonsteroidal anti-inflammatory drugs *(NSAIDs)*. A group of drugs having analgesic (pain relief), antipyretic (fever reducing), and anti-inflammatory effects.

Nonunion Failure of the ends of a fractured bone to unite.

Nuclear scintigraphy The production of two-dimensional images measuring the path of an internal radiopharmaceutical element. Commonly used in veterinary medicine to study skeletal structure, the liver, kidneys, and the thyroid.

Nutrition The intake of nutrients and their assimilation and utilization; provides energy, maintenance, and growth.

Oblique At a slant, angle, or incline; a radiographic position.

Olecranon The bony projection of the ulna at the elbow.

Open fracture A fracture in which a broken bone protrudes through the skin.

Open wounds A tissue, cavity, or lesion that is normally closed, but which injury has not yet healed.

Opiates A sedative narcotic containing opium or a derivative thereof.

Orthopedic The preservation and restoration of skeletal function, articulation, and structure. Correcting deformities (muscular and skeletal) through surgery.

Orthopedic Foundation for Animals (OFA)   A registry for dogs that have been radiographically examined for inherited orthopedic conditions (hips and elbows).

Ostectomy   Removal of a bone, or a portion thereof.

Osteitis   Inflammation of bone.

Osteoarthritis   A *non*inflammatory degenerative joint disease.

Osteoblasts   Cells (of mesenchymal origin) that produce bone.

Osteochondritis dissecans (OCD)   Inflammation of bone and cartilage resulting in the splitting of a piece of cartilage.

Osteochondrosis   Abnormal differentiation of growth cartilage.

Osteoclasts   Cells of bone marrow origin that resorb bone mineral and matrix.

Osteocyte   Cell within bone that originates from osteoblasts that become surrounded by and embedded in the bone they produce. Osteocytes retain minimal ability to produce bone.

Osteoid   Unmineralized bone matrix.

Osteolysis   Dissolving of bone, loss of calcium.

Osteomalacia   Softening of adult bone; causes pain, stiff gait, or lameness.

Osteomyelitis   Inflammation of bone marrow and adjacent bone.

Osteonecrosis   Necrosis (degeneration) of a bone.

Osteopenia   Bone mass reduced or decreased below normal.

Osteophytes   A bony outgrowth.

Osteophytosis   An abnormal increase of a bony outgrowth.

Osteoporosis   Bone with a loss of normal structure and lightened or porous condition.

Osteosarcoma   Malignant tumor of the bone producing cells, common in large-breed dogs.

Osteosynthesis   The surgical fastening of the ends of a fractured bone.

Osteotome   A bone knife, chisel shaped.

Osteotomy   Incision or transection of a bone.

Packed cell volume (PCV)   A sample volume of whole blood, centrifuged to allow measurement of the red blood cell volume percentage.

Palmar   The surface on the front paws that faces the ground. See Plantar.

Palpation   Examination of body parts by touch and feel.

Panosteitis   A self limiting spontaneous inflammation of the bone in young, large breed dogs.

Paralyzed   Loss of function or impairment of a nerve or muscle.

Parathyroid   Glands that regulate the absorption of calcium, located near the thyroid.

Pasteurella   A gram-negative anaerobic bacteria.

Patella   A large sesamoid bone in the stifle joint (kneecap).

Paw   Foot.

Pectineus muscle   A comb-like muscle on the medial thigh.

Pectineus tendon   The distal portion of the pectineus muscle attaching to the femur.

Pelvic   Pertaining to the pelvis.

Penrose drains   A tubular length of rubber anchored in a cavity or infected area to allow drainage for fluid or infected material.

Periarticular   Situated around a joint.

Periodontal disease   A disease or disorder of the tissues supporting the teeth.

Periosteum   Connective tissue covering all bones of the body. Fibrous and osteogenic membrane lining the exterior of the bone.

Periostitis   Inflammation of the periosteum.

Peripheral nerve disease   Injury or disease affecting a nerve outside the central nervous system.

Phagocytosis   Cellular action in which microorganisms are engulfed.

Phalanges   The bones of a digit or toe.

Phenylbutazone   A nonsteroidal, anti-inflammatory drug with analgesic or antipyretic properties.

Phosphorus   Essential nutrient in the diet; amount must be in proper ratio to calcium and other nutrients.

Physical therapy   Therapeutic methods to reduce pain, prevent disabilities, improve healing, and restore strength.

Physis (growth plate)   Area of the hyaline cartilage that lies between the epiphysis and metaphysis in growing animals.

Plantar   The surface on the rear paws that faces the ground.

Plasmacytic-lymphocytic synovitis   An immune-mediated inflammatory joint disease.

Plate   Metal implant used for fracture repairs.

Polyarthrodysplasia   Abnormality of development in multiple joints.

Polydactyly   The presence of extra digits; an inherited defect.

Polysulfated glycosaminoglycans   Adequan, a pharmaceutical to improve joint viscosity and reduce the pain of degenerative joint disease.

Popliteal tendon   The tendon behind the stifle.

Postoperative   After a surgical operation.

Prednisone   A cortisone derivative, with similar uses but greater potency.

Proprioceptive deficits   A deficiency of sensory nerves causing the dog to be unaware of limb placement or movement.

Prostaglandins   Control inflammation and vascular permeability in joints as well as other non orthopedic functions.

Protein synthesis Creation of new protein compounds from essential amino acids.

Proteins Essential nutrients, amino acids.

Proteoglycans Glycoproteins found in connective tissue.

Proximal The area closer to the main portion of a structure. When describing the limbs, this would be the ends attaching to the body trunk.

Pseudoarthrosis A nonosseous union of a fractured bone creating a false joint.

Pubis Part of the pelvic girdle.

Pyrexia A fever; elevated body temperature.

Quadriceps The combined term for four muscles of the cranial thigh.

Radial Pertaining to the radius of the lower forelimb.

Radiation therapy The treatment of cancer with megavoltage radiation to stop the further development of abnormal cells.

Radiography The imaging of body structures on x-ray film for diagnostic purposes.

Radius One of the two long bones of the forelimb, medial to the ulna.

Range of motion The degree to which a joint can be moved through extending and flexing.

Reconstruction Rebuilding of a structure by surgical correction.

Reduction Correction of a fracture or luxation with (open) or without (closed) a surgical incision to the site.

Reflex An involuntary action; reflexes are tested during a neurological examination.

Relaxation Lessening of tension.

Remodeling Reshaping of bone or other substance. May be done as a medical procedure or through regeneration/degeneration.

Renal function (Kidney function) A variety of tests are available to test various aspects of function.

Restraint Control of an animal by physical or chemical means.

Retrograde Moving backwards.

Rheumatoid arthritis An autoimmune disease that causes swelling or lameness in joints.

Rickettsia The cause of Rocky Mountain Spotted Fever; a microscopic parasite.

Robert Jones A heavily padded bandage for temporary support or pressure of a limb.

Rocky Mountain Spotted Fever An infectious disease caused by a microscopic parasite (rickettsii, transmitted by ticks).

Rotation The movement of a limb around its long axis or central line.

Sacroiliac   The joint of the sacrum and ilium; tail area of the back.

Salter-Harris fracture   A classification of fractures of the growth plate (physis).

Scapula   The shoulder blade.

Scapulohumeral   The joint of the scapula and humerus.

Scar tissue   A thick area of granulation tissue.

Sciatic nerve   A large nerve extending down the thigh from the lumbosacral region.

Screws   Used in placement of compression plates for fracture repair.

Septic arthritis   Used to designate arthritis of a joint that has a bacterial infection present.

Septicemia   Toxins (poisons) or microorganisms that have spread throughout the body's circulatory system.

Septum   A wall that separates body spaces or cavities.

Sequestration   An abnormal separation of a part from a whole.

Sequestrum   The section of dead tissue separated from healthy normal tissue.

Seroma   A collection of serum.

Serratus ventralis   A muscle connecting the scapula to the cervical vertebrae. It is essential in supporting the body trunk and in carrying the trunk and shoulder both forward and backward.

Serum chemistry profile   See Blood chemistry.

Shaft   The body, or straight portion, of the femur.

Shoulder   The joint formed by the humerus and scapula, a ball and socket joint.

Signalment   Description of a patient by using species, breed, sex, age, and weight as indicators.

Skeletal disease   An abnormality affecting the supporting structure of the body, i.e., orthopedic disease.

Skin   The largest organ of the body, a protective barrier against infection.

Skull   The bony framework of the head comprised of cranium and facial sections.

Slings   Suspension apparatus to support a body part (limb, body or tail).

Soft tissue   Body tissue that does not consist of bone or cartilage.

Spinal canal   The canal formed by the vertebrae, enclosing the spinal cord.

Spinal cord disease   A structure or function abnormality of the spinal cord.

Spinal cord lesions   A change in the spinal cord caused by trauma or pathology.

Spinal fractures   Usually a result of spinal trauma (auto accident, fighting, fall, or gunshot wound), they cause acute spinal cord compression.

Spongy bone   Spongiosa, the spongy internal substance of bone.

Spoon splints   Metasplint, a spoon-shaped splint made of heavy plastic or aluminum that offers support to the hind or front limb, especially the metatarsal region.

Sprains   Twisting or rupture of a joint or its ligaments.

Staphylococcus   A genus or family of gram-positive bacteria present on the skin and upper respiratory tract, a common cause of infection.

Steroids   Complex molecules that combine to form many important hormones, including male and female, adrenal, and sterols such as cholesterol.

Stifle   The knee, the joint of the femur, tibia, and patella.

Stifle arthrodesis   Surgical fusion of the stifle joint.

Strain   Overstretching of a muscle, overexertion.

Streptococcus   A genus of gram-positive aerobic bacteria.

Stress   A biological reaction to adverse conditions that disturb the organism, may lead to disease.

Subchondral   Below cartilage, usually describing a portion of bone.

Subluxation   A partial dislocation.

Subtrochanteric   The area below the trochanter, on the upper extremity and below the neck of the femur.

Supracondylar   Above any rounded part in the joint of some bones.

Swelling   An abnormal enlargement of a body part.

Synovial fluid   The clear fluid normally present in joint cavities, produced by the synovial membrane.

Synovial joint   Surrounds a body articulation (joint), allowing free movement of limbs.

Synovial membrane   The inner layer of the synovial joint, secretes synovial fluid.

Synovitis   Inflammation of the synovial membrane.

Systemic   Throughout the body or a body system.

T-plate   An orthopedic compression plate used in arthrodesis (a surgical fusion process) of the hock.

Tail   The end of the vertebral column, a caudal (body) appendage.

Talus   The tarsal bone (hock joint) of the hind limbs that connects with the tibia and fibula.

Tarsocrural joint   The area of the tarsal bones that connects with the tibia and fibula.

Tarsometatarsal joint   The area of the tarsus (hock) and metatarsus (rear pastern).

Tarsus   The hock joint.

Temporomandibular joint   The temporal (temple) bone of the cranium joining with the mandible (jaw).

Tendon   Connects muscle to a bone.

Tension   Putting pressure on a body part; stretching or straining.

Thoracic   Pertaining to the chest.

Thorax   The chest, between the neck and abdomen.

Tibia   The inner bone of the lower hind limb, between the stifle and hock.

Torsion   Twisted; may apply to skeletal structures or body organs.

Trabecular bone   (Spongy bone) Needle-shaped bone present in the marrow cavity.

Tranquilizer   A medication to calm or quiet anxiety.

Transverse   Crossing from one side to another.

Trauma   A wound or injury as a result of an external force.

Triceps   A muscle in the forelimb.

Trochanter   Pertaining to protrubences on the femur which are classified as greater, lesser and third.

Tumors   Lumps, neoplasms, abnormal new cell growths.

Ulcer   Usually thought associated with gastric conditions, may occur on any body organ or tissue, an excavation or defect in the normal surface.

Ulna   The medial bone next to the radius in the lower forelimb.

Uniaxial force   Force moving in a central direction *only*.

Ununited anconeal process   Elbow dysplasia; growth plate in elbow does not fuse.

Urinalysis   A laboratory analysis of urine to determine abnormal substances that may be present; a diagnostic test for various disease conditions.

Velocity   Rate of speed or movement of a body or a fluid within the body (i.e., relating to blood flowing through the heart chambers).

Ventral   The underside of the head, abdomen, and body; opposite the back.

Vertebra   A bony segment of the spine.

Vertical   Upright or a position perpendicular to a horizontal plane.

von Willebrands Disease   A genetic disease characterized by prolonged bleeding/coagulation time.

Walking   The slowest gait, observed as part of an orthopedic exam.

Weight   Measured in pounds or kilograms, body weight of an animal or amount of pressure or stress a support structure must endure.

Weight bearing   Analysis of weight supported by a limb.

White blood cell   Leukocyte, protects the body against infection.

Wound   Physical injury to the body.

Woven bone   Bone matrix deposited in a haphazard pattern so that the collagen fibers are somewhat randomly arranged.

Xenograft   A tissue graft transplantation between animals of different species.

Zygomatic bone   The bone extending from the cheek to the lateral rim over the eye.

BIBLIOGRAPHY

American Veterinary Medical Association. "Cancer in Animals." AVMA, Schaumburg, Illinois, 1987.

Corely, E. A., and G. G. Keller, *Hip Dysplasia, A Progress Report and Update.* Columbia, Missouri: The Orthopedic Foundation for Animals, 1993.

de LaHunta, Alexander. *Veterinary Neuroanatomy and Clinical Neurology.* 2nd ed. Philadelphia: W. B. Saunders Company, 1983.

Kealy, R. D., S. E. Olsson, K. L. Monti, D. F. Lawler, D. N. Biery, R. W. Helms, G. Lust, and G. K. Smith, "Effects of Limited Food Consumption on the Incidence of Hip Dysplasia in Growing Dogs." *JAVMA* 201[6]: 857-863 Sep 15 '92.

Mueller, Larry. "Miracle Cure for Hip Dysplasia?" *Outdoor Life* (January 1996): 27-32.

Olmstead, Marvin L. *Small Animal Orthopedics.* St. Louis: Mospby, 1994.

The Orthopedic Foundation for Animals. "Elbow Registry Update." OFA, Columbia, Missouri.

The Orthopedic Foundation for Animals. "Hip Registry." OFA, Columbia, Missouri.

The Orthopedic Foundation for Animals. "Warning, Is Your Dog at Risk to Develop Hip Dysplasia?" OFA, Columbia, Missouri.

Richardson, D. C., Mark Morris Associates, Topeka, Kansas. "The Role of Nutrition in Canine Hip Dysplasia." *Veterinary Clinics of North America, Small Animal Practice* 22 (1992): 529-540.

Smith GK, Biery DN, Gregor TP. New concepts of coxofemoral joint stability and the development of a clinical stress-radiographic method for quantitating hip joint laxity in the dog. *J Am Vet Med Assoc* 1990;196(1):59-70.

Smith GK and McKelvie PJ. Current concepts in the diagnosis of canine hip dysplasia, in Bonagura JD (ed): *Kirk's Current Veterinary Therapy XII: Small Animal Practice.* Philadelphia, WB Saunders, 1995.

Walkowicz and Wilcox, DVM. *Successful Dog Breeding.* 2nd ed. New York: Howell Book House, 1994.

Whittick, William G. *Canine Orthopedics.* 2nd ed. Philadelphia: Lea and Febifer, 1990.

INDEX

Myasthenia gravis
  breeds prone to, 22, 23, 26
  description of, 152
Myelography
  of cauda equina syndrome, 146
  of hypoplasia of dens, 147
  of intervertebral disk disease, 141
  of spinal cord/vertebral column
    lesions, 215-16
  of Wobblers Syndrome, 143

N

Naproxen, 195-96
Neck palpation, 66
Neoplasias, 154-57, 213
  breeds prone to, 22, 23, 24, 25,
    26, 27, 28, 29
Neostigmine (Prostigmin), 152
Neuromuscular stimulation,
  197-98
Neurotropic osteopathy, 23
Neutering, 161, 238-39
Newfoundlands, 25, 75, 101, 105,
  115
Non-Sporting dogs, 28-29
Nonsteroidal anti-inflammatory drugs
  (NSAIDs), 146, 193, 194-96, 197
Nutritional secondary
  hyperparathyroidism, 151-52

O

Oblique fractures, 204
Obstacle course (exercise), 61
Old English Sheepdogs, 13, 29, 146,
  158
Open fractures, 165, 203
Open technique, 205
Opioids, 72
Orthopedic Foundation for Animals
  (OFA), 18, 75-76, 95, 101-2, 173,
  175
Osteoarthritis, 66
  clinical signs of, 121
  hip dysplasia and, 91, 97

intertrochanteric osteotomy and,
  220
pectineus tendonectomy and, 221
pelvic osteotomy and, 218, 219
total hip replacement and, 222
Osteoarthrosis, see Osteoarthritis
Osteochondritis dissecans (OCD),
  80-83
  of the hock, 83
  breeds prone to, 22, 23, 24, 25, 29
  case report of, 50-51
  of the elbow, 82
  of the shoulder, 80-82
  of the stifle, 82
  surgical repair procedures for,
    81-82, 200-2
Osteochondrosis, 76
  description of, 79-80
  of the spine, 23, 24
Osteodystrophy, 23
Osteogenesis imperfecta, 28
Osteomyelitis, 167
Osteopenia, 27, 149, 150-54
Osteoporosis, 22, 24, 35
Osteosarcomas, 155, 198
Otterhounds, 24

P

Pain, see also Analgesic therapy
  acute, 192
  chronic, 192
  deep, 133, 134
  generalized, 192
Painted toenails (exercise), 61
Palpation, 62
  in elbow dysplasia diagnosis,
    65-66, 93-94
  in hip dysplasia diagnosis, 66-67,
    91-93
  of knees, 68-69, 109
  of neck, 66
  of shoulder, 63-65
Pannus, 22, 29
  atypical, 27, 28
Panosteitis, 23, 29, 85, 86f

Q - R